Nursing Administration Review and Resource Manual, 2nd Ed.

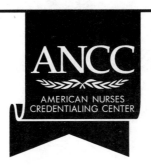

D1456453

10/07

ISBN 10: 0-9768213-9-7
ISBN 13: 978-0-9768213-9-7

Nursing Administration Review and Resource Manual, 2nd Ed.

December 2006

Please direct your comments and/or queries to:
revmanuals@ana.org

The health care services delivery system is a volatile marketplace demanding superior knowledge, clinical skills, and competencies from all registered nurses. Nursing autonomy of practice, and nurse career marketability and mobility in the new century hinge on affirming the profession's formative philosophy which places a priority on a lifelong commitment to the principles of education and professional development. The knowledge base of nursing theory and practice is expanding, and while care has been taken to ensure the accuracy and timeliness of the information presented in the **Nursing Administration Review and Resource Manual,** clinicians are advised to always verify the most current national treatment guidelines and recommendations and to practice in accordance with professional standards of care used with regard to the unique circumstances that apply in each practice situation. In addition, every effort has been made in this text to insure accuracy and, in particular to confirm that drug selections and dosages are in accordance with current recommendations and practice, including the ongoing research, changes to government regulations and the developments in product information provided by pharmaceutical manufacturers. However, it is the responsibility of each nurse practitioner to verify drug product information and to practice in accordance with professional standards of care. In addition, the editors wish to note that provision of information in this text does not imply an endorsement of any particular products, procedures or services. As a review text, this content is provided at a level that describes what a FNP should know upon entry into practice. NPs may object, for religious or other reasons, to the provisions of certain services. That decision, too, must be left to the individual NP.

Therefore, the authors, editors, American Nurses Association (ANA), American Nurses Association's Publishing (ANP), American Nurses Credentialing Center (ANCC), and the Institute for Credentialing Innovation cannot accept responsibility for errors or omissions, or for any consequences or liability, injury and/or damages to persons or property from application of the information in this manual and make no warranty, express or implied, with respect to the contents of the **Nursing Administration Review and Resource Manual.**

Published by:

The Institute for Credentialing Innovation
8515 Georgia Avenue, Suite 400
Silver Spring, MD 20910-3402
www.nursecredentialing.org

The American Nurses Credentialing Center would like to acknowledge the editors, contributors and reviewers who assisted in development of the first edition of the Nursing Administration Review and Resource Manual

Lynne Baker, MS, RN, CNA, Author
Bessie Marquis, MSN, RN, Contributing Author

Table of Contents

Introduction

Welcome! This review program provides a practical overview of the subject matter included in the American Nurses Credentialing Center's (ANCC) certification examinations in nursing administration. ANCC offers two levels of nursing administration certification: 1) Nursing Administration (Exam #10) for those at the manager level and Nursing Administration; 2) Advanced (Exam #11) for those at the executive level. As nursing administration expands beyond the traditional setting of the hospital, so too does the nurse executive's knowledge base need to widen to incorporate the larger universe of health care.

This course is a synthesis and revision of earlier nursing administration certification review programs compiled over the years. The contributions of those who have gone before is gratefully acknowledged.

The course is constructed in outline form consistent with the major subjects covered in the certification examinations. The content is meant to reinforce the reader's current understanding about key issues in the field of nursing administration rather than to implant new knowledge. The major topic areas are:

- Organization and Structure
- Economics
- Human Resources
- Ethics
- Legal and Regulatory Issues

The information in this study guide was constructed consistent with the approach used by the American Nurses Credentialing Center in creating its nursing administration certification examinations. It is intended as a "quick review" for nurse managers and administrators who are already skillful leaders and who daily put into practice the concepts and theories outlined above.

CHAPTER 1

Organization and Structure

THEORIES

Organizational

The classical principles of organizational structure include chain of command, unity of command, and span of control. In today's dynamic business environment, these principles are challenged in practice if not in theory.

- **Chain of command** implies that there is an unbroken line of command from the top to the bottom of the organization. Each unit within the organization is connected to another. Hypothetically, reporting relationships are constrained by the chain of command with each subsequent "layer" reporting administratively to the one immediately above it. In a positive sense, the chain of command insures a smooth exchange of information from top to bottom and vice versa. In practice, the feedback loops necessary to assure that upward as well as downward messages are heard and understood are at times absent.
- **Unity of command** holds that each subordinate is accountable to only one superior. Expectations are clearly defined and well understood.
- **Span of control** defines the scope of responsibility of a given supervisor/manager. Theoretically, tasks and responsibilities are divided so that goals are accomplished without undue burden on any one person or unit within the organization.
- **Organizational charts** reflect the principles noted above, with each person or unit connected to another, generally in a hierarchical fashion. The extent to which organizational charts reflect actual behavior within organizations is questionable. Nonetheless, organizational charts do clarify relationships between and among people and functions within organizations and can be used to profile any of a variety of organizational structures. Organizational charts show formal relationships, but not informal or informational connections among people or groups in organizations. Thus, they may show structure as it is assumed to be, not as it is. Organizational charts are labeled to illustrate how services are arranged within an establishment, for example, service line (neurology, endocrinology, oncology); geography (4 West, 4 South, 6 North); service delivery (Intensive Care, Transitional Care Unit, Orthopedic Surgery). Organizational charts may also reflect the manner in which the organization operates, in other words, functional, matrix.

Management

Management, much like nursing, is considered both art and science. The "aim" of management is to create a surplus; that is, to establish an environment in which people can accomplish their goals with the least amount of time, money, materials, and personal dissatisfaction, or where they can achieve as much as possible of a desired goal with available resources. Management came into its own in the industrial age when guilds, crafts, and agriculture gave way to mass production and specialization. Management was, and is, seen as a means to accomplish an intended outcome through the work of others.

The traditional functions of management are these:

- Plan — decide in advance what to do, how to do it, when to do it and who is to do it;
- Organize — establish an intentional structure of roles; assume that all tasks necessary to accomplish goals are assigned to people who can perform the task(s);
- Staff — fill positions and keep them filled;
- Lead — influence people so that they willingly and enthusiastically work to achieve the goals of the organization;
- Control — measure and correct activities of subordinates to assure conformance to plans;
- Coordinate — achieve harmony of individual efforts in order to achieve intended goals.

Management Theories and Theorists

Scientific Management

Fredrick Taylor is considered the "father" of scientific management. His era spans the late nineteenth and early twentieth centuries and the beginning of industrialization. His contemporaries include Frank and Lillian Gilbreth, Henry Gantt, Harrington Emerson, and Morris Cook. The major concept underlying the work of Taylor and his colleagues is that of *efficiency*. Efficiencies were created through the establishment of standards, time-motion studies, task analysis, job simplification, and productivity incentives.

Process Management

Henry Fayol is the champion of the management process school that came into vogue following World War I and during the Great Depression (early twentieth century into the 1930s). Others whose work is associated with this era include Max Weber, James Mooney, and Lyndall Urwick.

The process school looked at the whole of an organization, not merely at its parts. Competency rather than favoritism was seen as a driver. Rules were established to govern practice and workers could expect to be adequately compensated.

Administratively, hierarchy prevailed, with clear delineation of one's authority based on the assigned position within the organization's traditional pyramidal structure. Authority to direct the activities of others flowed downward level by level. The "universal" principles of management—span of control, chain of command, accountability, and responsibility, planning, organizing, coordinating, and controlling—were defined during this era.

Human Relations Management

The 1940s were a time of relative prosperity in the United States. Middle-class values predominated, the working class became more educated, and managers were able to focus attention on interpersonal relationships within the workplace. Harvard researchers Elton Mayo and Fritz Roethlisberger conducted the Hawthorne Shirt Factory studies during this time. The Western Electric Company wanted to investigate the influence of working conditions on employee efficiency and productivity. Although working conditions, specifically the level of light, were manipulated as part of the research design, the investigators found no correlation between workers' productivity and the condition of the environment. They did conclude that workers performed differently when they were being observed. Even today, the "Hawthorne effect" is frequently cited to explain the significance of relationships between managers and frontline workers relative to business outcomes, either positive or negative. While the validity and reliability of the Hawthorne study itself can be called into question, the term has taken its place in the management lexicon. Cooperation between labor and management, democratization of the workplace (in contrast to autocracy), and the criticality of communication are among the concepts that define this period.

Behavioral Science and Management

Abraham Maslow and Fredrick Herzberg are associated with the behavioral school that gained prominence in the 1950s. Douglas MacGregor, Chris Argyris, Rensis Likert, Robert Blake, Jane Mouton, Paul Hersey, Fred Fiedler, and Kenneth Blanchard also gained distinction during this time. Their names and their work are likely to be familiar to many readers of this study guide. Indeed, a number of their writings are considered management classics and some have found a place in popular literature as well as in the academic arena. *The One Minute Manager* (Blanchard) and related spin-offs come to mind.

The behaviorists built on the work began during the "human relations" period. Concepts that took shape during this time include:

- Hierarchy of needs, which hold that the needs of one level must be satisfied before one can advance to the next level;
- Personal motivators and hygiene factors are complementary and of equal importance;
- Workers need to have a say in operations; self-direction results in satisfaction;
- Leadership style is important; participative management is the preferred mode.

The workforce during this era was relatively homogenous, fairly prosperous, and better educated. More women assumed jobs outside the home. Many women entered the workforce as a matter of national necessity during the war years; some stayed, though in jobs different than those they held during the 1940s.

Management by Objectives

Peter Drucker and George Odiorne spearheaded the management by objectives (MBO) movement during the 1970s and 1980s; their concepts remain viable in the current era. Increasing conservatism, a focus on the bottom line, personal accountability, and an emphasis on standards characterize the MBO philosophy. Business schools came into their own and the number of college graduates increased significantly.

Total Quality Management and Continuous Quality Improvement

Edwards Deming, Joseph Juran, and Phil Crosby are the recognized leaders in the total quality (TQM) and continuous quality (CQI) arena. Though Deming's and Juran's work progressed quietly during the post-World War II years, it was conducted mostly in Japan. TQM/CQI did not gain popularity in the United States until the 1980s and 1990s in the wake of the realization that merchandise produced in Japan was often superior to and less expensive than goods produced elsewhere, including the United States. Examined more closely, the principles that underlie TQM/CQI are those of the scientific method conveyed in ways that generated acceptance by business leaders in the United States.

The contributions of Walter Shewhart, the father of statistical quality control, are sometimes overlooked in the popularization of TQM/CQI. It was Shewhart who successfully brought together the disciplines of statistics, engineering, and economics and became known as the father of modern quality control. The lasting and tangible evidence of that union—for which he is most widely known—is the simple but highly effective tool known as the control chart.

"Systems thinking," popularized by Peter Senge and his colleagues from Massachusetts Institute of Technology (MIT) in *The Fifth Discipline,* grew out of the TQM/CQI movement. These concepts have moved into the health care realm under the guidance of physicians Donald Berwick and Paul Batalden and the Institute for Healthcare Improvement.

The Joint Commission on the Accreditation of Healthcare Organizations (JCAHO) adopted TQM/CQI and has built the principles into its requirements. Concepts that form the foundation of TQM/CQI include benchmarking, statistical process control, reduction of variation, application of the Pareto Principle (focus on the "vital few" rather than the "trivial many"), application of the plan-do-check-act (PDCA) cycle to achieve systems improvement, systems modification in contrast to personal blame, the use of teams, and a focus on meeting customer needs.

Over time, the manager's role has changed from that of overseer and controller to one of coach and supporter. Characteristics of the modern manager include: a belief that people are basically "good" (trustworthy) and capable of change, an appreciation of the value of diversity in contrast to homogeneity, an awareness that power shared is power gained, creative use of conflict in contrast to avoidance of dissension at all cost, risk taking in contrast to risk aversion, and fostering collaboration rather than competition (particularly among staff who must work together to get the job done).

Nursing

As with management, nursing has undergone changes throughout the years in response to societal needs and professional reasoning. The Great Depression, World War II, cyclic nursing shortages, and economics all played a role in modifying nursing's pathway. Prior to the Depression of the late 1920s and early 1930s, nurses in the field of public health in particular enjoyed relative independence in practice and commanded respect within the medical community. Their basic education took place in an academic setting instead of in a hospital environment. With a background in epidemiology as well as in patient care, they were on the forefront of community-based care systems. The anticipated trajectory was interrupted with the severe economic downturn of the Depression and cutbacks in funding for highly effective nurse-managed programs. Though academic programs in nursing survived, the recommendations of the Brown Report, issued in 1923, were not adopted, and the primary learning environment for nurses remained that of the hospital setting.

The early "modern" era of nursing found nursing students in what some might call a "servant role," in that student nurses provided much of the care to hospitalized patients in return for the clinical education accompanied by "board and room." The students were almost exclusively young women, newly graduated from high school, unmarried, and committed to a career of service.

When World War II loomed on the horizon, registered nurses were called to serve in the military, leaving a noticeable gap in the workforce even as more people were being cared for in the hospital setting. To fill the gap, the "practical nurse" role came into being as a hypothetically temporary solution to that era's nursing shortage. An abbreviated curriculum was created to prepare practical nurses to assume designated bedside duties, thereby freeing the registered nurses remaining in the private sector to become overseers of care more than direct caregivers. Through the legislative process, practical nurses were eventually able to sit for an examination and become licensed as LPNs or LVNs (licensed practical nurse or licensed vocational nurse). The role of the nurse's aide also came into being during this time to fill the need for caregivers. Most nurse's aides learned their trade on the job. Over the years, more formal nurse's aide training programs have been developed and are generally offered through adult learning or vocational training programs.

As nursing has taken on an increasingly professional mantle, so, too, have models of care evolved. The common thread among all models is that of the nursing process. The elements of the nursing process are assessment, planning, intervention, and evaluation. In other words, the scientific process that also forms the basis for modern management.

1

Nursing Theory

Nursing theory is a relatively recent construct, with most theory development taking place in the 1960s, 1970s, and beyond. However, nursing historians and researchers acknowledge that Nightingale's "environmental factors" concept fits the definition of descriptive theory. Nightingale held that nurses did not need to be fully versed in the disease model in order to fashion a therapeutic environment. Rather, she demonstrated that fresh air, light, cleanliness, adequate nutrition, and quietness fostered healing and wellness. Her assertions about the body's "reparative processes" provided her students with a way to think about their practice as a distinct entity, not merely as an extension of medicine. She is also credited with applying statistics to the field of health care well in advance of the era when such practice became common.

Nursing owes a debt of gratitude to a handful of nursing educators who took their master's and doctoral degrees in education from the University of Columbia Teachers' College and then became pioneers in the design of theory-based curricula for the field of nursing. Peplau, Henderson, Hall, Abdellah, King, Wiedenbach, and Rogers are among the early Columbia graduates whose names are associated with modern theories of nursing. In the mid-1970s, the National League for Nursing (NLN) made theory-based nursing a requirement for accreditation.

Nursing theory continues to evolve, as does the definition of nursing. The most recent iteration of the definition, first published in 1980, is articulated in the 2003 edition of *Nursing's Social Policy Statement* (ANA, 2003). It states, "nursing is the prevention of illness, the alleviation of suffering and the protection, promotion and restoration of heath in the care of individuals, families, groups, communities and populations." The *Social Policy Statement* reinforces the assertion that nursing practice embraces four essential components: attention to the full range of human experience, integration of objective and subjective phenomena, application of scientific knowledge, and provision of care that fosters health and healing. Brief sketches of several theories of nursing that reinforce nursing's intent are presented below. The list is not all-inclusive.

The focus of Hildegard Peplau's work (1952) was on the interactive processes that form the basis of the nurse-client relationship. The nurse serves as resource, counselor, and surrogate. The relationship between client and nurse is progressive and overlapping and proceeds through these phases: orientation, identification, explanation, and resolution.

Virginia Henderson (1955, 1964) saw nursing as embracing the whole person and defines the practice as "assisting the individual, sick or well, in the performance of those activities contributing to health or its recovery (or to peaceful death) that he would perform unaided if he had the necessary strength, will or knowledge. And to do this in such a way as to help him gain independence as rapidly as possible."

Consistent with her definition, Henderson described the role of the nurse as substitutive (doing for the person), supplementary (helping the person), or complementary (working with the person), with the goal of helping the person become as independent as possible. She categorized nursing functions into fourteen components based on meeting human needs, for example, breathing, eating/drinking, elimination, worship, work, and so forth.

As did Henderson, Faye Abdellah (1960) defined nursing as meeting the needs of the whole person— physical, emotional, intellectual, social, and spiritual. The nurse assumes responsibility for the care of the family as well as that of the client (patient). S/he is problem solver and decision maker and formulates a plan of care that includes four dimensions: comfort; hygiene and safety; physiological balance; psychological and social factors; and community and sociological factors. Abdellah identified twenty-one nursing problems, which, if addressed by the nurse, lead to improvement in the client's status.

Ida Orlando (1961) focused on the nurse's response to the immediate need of the client in a given situation. The situation is characterized by these three elements: client behavior, nurse reaction, and nurse actions. Once the nurse identifies the client's need, s/he acts "automatically or deliberatively" to meet the need and in so doing reduces the distress experienced by the client.

Myra Levine (1973) saw the client as someone who interacts with and adapts to his environment. Conservation of energy is a primary concern and it is nursing's role to assist the client to conserve his/her "resources" to promote health. Levine's four conservation principles of nursing are: 1) conservation of client energy; 2) conservation of structural integrity; 3) conservation of personal integrity; 4) conservation of social integrity.

Dorothy Johnson (1968) proposed that nursing's role is to relieve illness-induced stress so that the client is more easily able to regain equilibrium and proceed through recovery. The nurse focuses on seven areas of behavior (behavioral subsystems) and intervenes to reestablish balance in any or all of the systems under stress as a means of restoring health.

Martha Rogers (1970) took nursing's theoretical framework to a new level by asserting that the human organism is an energy field in a constant state of change, coexisting in the universe; in other words, human beings are part of the universe and as such influence and are influenced by the environment that surrounds them and of which they are in integral part. Rogers viewed nursing as "humanistic science" and focused on the research aspects of the field.

Dorothy Orem (1971) embraced a philosophy of self-care and theorized that nursing's role is to intervene when the client is unable to fulfill her biological, psychological, developmental, or social needs. The nurse is responsible for determining why a client is unable to meet her needs in the listed dimensions and then intervenes to help the client regain her ability to provide self-care in any or all dimensions.

Betty Neuman's theory (1972) is based on a holistic perspective that sees human beings as part of an "open system"; they are in a state of constant adjustment as they interact with, adjust to, and are adjusted by the environment. Neuman identified three categories of stressors that disrupt the system: intrapersonal (within the self), interpersonal (occurring between persons), and extrapersonal (occurring outside the person; e.g., financial stressors). Since nursing is concerned with restoring balance, the nurse's role is one of "systems management." Nursing actions are seen as preventative and are categorized by level: primary (identify risk factors and strengthen defenses), secondary (strengthen internal defenses by identifying priorities and establishing treatment plans), and tertiary (educate to prevent recurrence).

1

Callista Roy's adaptation model (1976 with subsequent revision and expansion) holds that people are co-extensive with their physical and social environments and that nursing's role is to enhance the well-being of the patient (person) and, by extension, the well-being of the earth ("cosmic unity"). The nurse identifies those demands that are causing problems for the client, determines how well the client is adapting to the demands, and provides care to help the client adapt more successfully. Roy proposes that all individuals must adapt to the following demands: 1) meeting basic physiological needs; 2) developing a positive self-concept; 3) performing social roles; 4) achieving balance between dependence and independence.

Madeleine Leininger's transcultural theory (1978) identified caring as the central focus and unifying domain of nursing. Transcultural nursing focuses on comparative study and analysis of different cultures and subcultures throughout the world with respect to their caring interventions, health-illness values, and patterns of behavior. The outcome is the development of a body of knowledge, both scientific and humanistic, from which to derive culture-specific and culture-universal nursing care practices.

Jean Watson (1979) reiterated that nursing is concerned with health promotion, health restoration, and prevention of illness, and that these ends are achieved through the integration of science and philosophy on the part of nurses, whose interpersonal interventions are designed to meet human needs.

Kathy Kolcaba's comfort theory (1991) embraced a concept with a strong association to nursing. Nurses traditionally provide comfort to patients and their families through interventions that can be called comfort measures. The intentional comforting actions of nurses usually are comforting to patients. Enhanced comfort, as an immediate desirable outcome of nursing care, is theoretically and positively correlated with desirable health seeking behaviors (HSBs). HSBs can be internal (healing, immune function, number of T cells, etc.), external (health-related activities, functional outcomes, hospital length of stay, hospital readmissions, etc.), or a peaceful death. The relationship between comfort and health-seeking behaviors are clarified in Kolcaba's comfort theory.

Change Theory

Maslow, Lewin, and Herzberg are names associated with the motivational theories that underlie popularly referenced change models. Maslow's hierarchy of needs and Herzberg's two-factor theory are contrasted in table 1–1 (adapted from Schermerhorn, Hunt, and Osborn, 2002).

Kurt Lewin proposed that individuals maintain the status quo or a state of equilibrium by balancing both driving and restraining forces operating within any field. He maintains that, for any change to occur, this balance must be disrupted. One must either increase the force of the driving forces or lessen the power of the restraining forces. Conventional wisdom holds that it is generally easier, or more productive, to decrease the power of the restraining force, to decrease resistance, than to strengthen the driving forces. Lewin also suggested that the steps in the change process are predictable. The steps are freezing, movement, and refreezing. Here are some of the components associated with Lewin's phases of change.

1

- Unfreezing
  - Gather data.
  - Diagnose the problem.
  - Decide if there is a need for change.
  - Make others aware of the need.
  - Confirm motivation for the change.
  - Proceed to step two (movement) only after the status quo has been sufficiently disrupted and there is a perceived need for change on the part of others.
- Movement
  - Develop plan.
  - Set goals and objectives.
  - Identify areas of support and resistance.
  - Include all who will be affected by the change in planning for the change.
  - Set target dates.
  - Develop change strategies.
  - Implement change.
  - Support and encourage others through the change.
  - Employ tactics designed to overcome resistance.
  - Evaluate the change.
  - Modify the change if necessary.

TABLE 1-1
Comparison of Maslow and Herzberg Theories

Hierarchy of Needs Theory		Two-Factor Theory
Self-actualization	Motivators	• Challenging work • Achievement • Growth in job • Responsibility
Esteem of status		• Advancement • Recognition • Status
Affiliation or acceptance	Maintenance Factors	• Interpersonal relations • Company policy and administration • Quality of supervision
Security or safety		• Quality of supervision • Working conditions • Job security
Physiological needs		• Salary • Personal life

1

- Refreezing
  - Change is integrated into the structure of the organization.
  - Support is in place to sustain the change.

Everett Rogers's research regarding the diffusion of innovation deserves mention in any dialogue about change. Here, greatly simplified, are a few of Rogers's concepts:

- Innovations that are perceived by individuals as having greater relative advantage and less complexity will be adopted more rapidly than other innovations.
- Adopter categories have been defined on the basis of innovativeness and more or less fall into a bell-shaped curve:
  - Innovators (2.5%): these are the risk takers; they are adventurous, independent, constantly seek information, generally have the means (finances, connections, etc.) to be "out in front." The opinion of others is not particularly relevant to innovators.
  - Early adopters (13.5%): translate the innovator's message for the early majority. They establish momentum for change and are respected opinion leaders.
  - Early majority (34%): deliberate, adopt new ideas just before the average member of a system; do not seek information on their own but are willing to hear and act on the message from the early adopters.
  - Late majority (34%): skeptical, adopt new ideas just after the average member of a system. They respond to the pressure of peers and then change accordingly. Their restraint is important in the change process in that they provide the provocative voice that sometimes moderates the rate of change or influences the change agents to use alternative tactics.
  - Resistors (16%): traditional, last in a social system to adopt an innovation; pay little attention to the opinions of others. The dissident voice, such as that of the resistor, is of value in any major change effort.

To understand the practical application of Rogers' work, one need only to look at the adoption of the Internet as an accepted way of doing business, gathering information, or learning.

The rapidity with which change is adopted and sustained in an organization has much to do with leadership's understanding of the complexity of the change process. Only if the actual or perceived threat is of such magnitude that maintaining the status quo is tantamount to disaster can massive change occur quickly and throughout an entire organization. Even then, there will be some who find it impossible to change. In many cases, these people will leave, or will be asked to leave, the organization. Connor (1995) terms the need for large-scale change in the midst of crisis the "burning platform" scenario.

Role

The role of the organization is to effectively use the resources at its command to achieve a predetermined outcome.

Leadership

The four leadership theories outlined here—trait, behavioral, contingency, and contemporary—have evolved over time and overlap to some extent.

Trait Theory

Leaders are assumed to possess certain traits that, if put into practice, result in success. Trait theory focuses on the characteristics of the leader. Stogdill is credited with identifying the initial set of leadership traits, which include drive, persistence, creative problem solving, initiative, self-confidence, acceptance of the consequences of one's actions, resilience, tolerance, ability to influence others, and ability to structure social interactions. The list was further expanded to include such traits as intelligence, integrity, nonconformity, cooperativeness, and tact.

Behavioral Theory

In contrast to the characteristics that leaders possess (trait theory), what leaders do, or how they behave, is the focus of behavioral theorists (see also the notes above under organizational theory, specifically the work of Maslow, Herzberg, and their contemporaries).

The behaviorists categorize leaders by their style of practice. **Autocratic** leaders purport to change the behavior of subordinates through external control with the use of coercion, authority, punishment, and power. In contrast, the **democratic** leader appeals to the drive of her/his subordinates and influences change through participation, involvement of subordinates in goal setting, and collaboration. The permissive or **laissez-faire** leader uses a "hands-off" approach and assumes people are able to make their own decisions and complete their work unaided by direction or facilitation. **Bureaucratic** leaders rely on organizational policies and rules to influence the behavior of their subordinates. Autocratic and bureaucratic leaders assume that external motivators cause subordinates to change their behavior. Democratic and laissez-faire leaders believe that behavior change is internally inspired (internal locus of control).

In order to demonstrate the effectiveness of various styles of leadership, Likert (Bateman and Snell, 2002) devised a four-quadrant model, known as System 4 Management, to illustrate the relationship between leadership behavior and outcomes. He describes leadership style according to the degree of involvement in decision making the manager invites from her/his subordinates. The terms Likert uses

1

are similar to those noted above: autocratic, benevolent, consultative, and partici-pative (democratic). His work shows that greater employee involvement translates to greater commitment to the organization and its objectives. The managerial grid developed by Blake and his colleagues (Bateman and Snell, 2002) is similar to Likert's quadrants and focuses on the varying degrees of concern the manager has for production, people, or both. For example, in Blake's schematic, the "impover-ished" leader has a low concern for both people and production, while the "team" manager shows high concern in both of these dimensions.

Contingency Theory

While leaders may have an affinity for a particular style, no one style works effective-ly in every situation. For example, a leader who employees a democratic style under conditions of stability may switch to an autocratic style in the face of an emergency that demands he/she take charge of the situation in order to achieve the best outcome. This ability to adapt one's approach to the situation at hand is labeled contingency theory, or situational leadership.

Fiedler (Schermerhorn, Hunt, and Osborn, 2002) describes three leadership fac-tors that influence outcomes:

- Manager-follower relationships — to what degree does the manager enjoy the loyalty and support of her/his subordinates?
- Task structure — to what degree is the task clearly described or the operating procedures in place to guarantee a successful outcome?
- Position power — to what degree is the manager able to administer rewards and punishment?

As an example, if a change in staffing practice is under consideration, it will have a better chance of acceptance if the leader-follower relationship is good, the task is structured, and the leader has high position power.

Hersey and Blanchard (Schermerhorn, Hunt, and Osborn, 2002) took Fiedler's model a step further and added followers' willingness and readiness. They recom-mend that leaders consider the *job maturity* and *psychological maturity* of their employees before deciding whether task performance or maintenance (relationship) behaviors on their part are more important. Job maturity refers to the employee's skill and technical knowledge relative to the job; psychological maturity refers to the employee's self-confidence and self-respect. Hersey and Blanchard posit that the leader, under the situational leadership model, uses these modes to move the agenda:

- Leadership Style S1 — High Task/Low Relationship (Telling) — the leader tells the worker what to do and provides close supervision;
- Leadership Style S2 — High Task/High Relationship (Selling) — the leader makes decisions and coaches followers; the leader provides opportunity for clar-ification;
- Leadership Style S3 — Low Task/High Relationship (Participating) — both leader and follower participate in projects and decisions;
- Leadership Style S4 — Low Task/Low Relationship (Delegating) — the leader gives subordinates the freedom to make decisions and carry out plans.

In addition, subordinate readiness occurs along a continuum from low to high relative to ability and willingness. For example, the employee may be categorized as:

- R1 — Unable and unwilling; insecure;
- R2 — Unable but willing; confident;
- R3 — Able but unwilling; insecure
- R4 — Able and willing; confident.

Vroom and Yetton's (Schermerhorn, Hunt, and Osborn, 2002) expectancy model offers a prescriptive approach for managers to use when determining the amount of participation they should solicit from employees. The manager will adjust her/his leadership style in a given situation once answers to three key questions are clear. The questions are:

- Is all the information available to make the decision?
- Is staff acceptance of the decision necessary to effective implementation?
- Would the group's decision be one the leader could live with?

According to this model, the manager will then choose one of five decision-making approaches: tell, sell, consult, join, or delegate.

Contemporary Theories

Newer concepts of leadership are an amalgam of prior work in the field and include such descriptors as charismatic, transactional, transformational, connective, shared, and servant leadership. The complexity of today's work environment demands flexibility and adaptability on the part of the leader as never before. There is no one "right" style of leadership.

Charismatic leaders are those who have the ability to engage others because of the power of their personalities. They inspire affection and emotional connection and may use the power of their personalities to advance revolutionary ideas.

Transactional leadership is derived from the principles of social-exchange theory. Social exchange implies that there are social, political, and psychological benefits to be had in any relationship, including that of leader and follower, and that these benefits are reciprocal. Both the manager and the employee derive equal benefit from their relationship and the interactions between them are meant to achieve and maintain balance (i.e., the status quo).

By contrast, transformational leadership moves people well beyond current reality. It seeks to gain support for change that is characterized as revolutionary. The leader is able to inspire others, to instill in them the belief that they can accomplish extraordinary things, often for the good of society.

Connective leadership draws on the leader's ability to bring others together as a means of effecting change. Leaders in this category realize that the whole is greater than the sum of its parts and achieve results through collaboration, cooperation, coordination, and collegiality. They are able to foster interconnectedness among seemingly disparate groups, are characterized as bridge builders, and are able to overcome the obstacles posed by hierarchical structures.

1

Shared leadership is based on the concept of empowerment. It recognizes the significance of informal as well as formal leadership to the success of any enterprise. It acknowledges that no one person can possibly possess all the knowledge or power needed to accomplish intended goals or outcomes within the organization. Self-directed work teams and shared governance epitomize the philosophy of shared leadership.

Servant leadership puts other people and their needs before the leader's self-interest. The person who chooses to serve may be called upon to lead and in so doing may transform the lives of her/his followers.

Decision Making
(see also Human Resources, Management Issues)

The "rational" model of decision making in organizations is no longer considered the only option. A concept termed "bounded reality" is probably more reasonable in that the assumptions of the rational model rarely hold true in organizational life. Bounded reality, a term coined by Nobel laureate Herbert Simon (Bateman and Snell, 2020), holds that leaders in organizations cannot make perfectly rational decisions because 1) they have imperfect and incomplete information about alternatives and consequences; 2) they face highly complex problems; 3) they cannot process all the information that confronts them (human capacity); 4) they do not have sufficient time to fully process the information that confronts them; and 5) they are faced with conflicting goals among the constituents of the organization.

Systems

Systems Theory

The theoretical construct underlying systems holds that systems are composed of interrelated parts and that the arrangement of the parts results in a unified whole. Systems can be "closed" or "open." Closed systems are assumed to occur only in the physical sciences (e.g., the circulatory system). Open systems interact internally and with the environment.

Organizations are defined as complex, sociotechnical open systems. "Parts" of the system are labeled as input, throughput, and output. Input is comprised of such elements as staff, patients, materials, financial resources, supplies, and equipment. Throughput is the process that is performed to create a product. Output is the *product*; within the health care system, it may be defined as restored health, dignified death, research, education, and so forth.

While systems theory provides a useful language to describe organizational operations, it falls short when attempting to identify, let alone describe, the numerous variables at work throughout the input–process-output (IPO) process (Schermerhorn, Hunt, and Osborn, 2002).

MISSION AND PHILOSOPHY

Purpose

The mission statement of an organization provides a general statement about its reason for existence (purpose). Its vision statement describes its aspiration(s), the goal(s) it wishes to achieve. The mission and vision statements of an organization are meant to inspire and motivate those associated with it. Both statements are relatively brief and precede the goals, objectives, and strategies of the establishment.

The mission statement flows from the organization's foundations. Does the organization have a social or community commitment? Does it have an educational affiliation? Who does it exist to serve? What is the scope of services it provides? Questions such as these should be answered in the few brief sentences that comprise the mission statement.

Mission statements are future oriented and speak to what an organization intends to achieve, given the resources at its disposal. Though idealistic, mission statements are created with the belief that what is promised is indeed attainable within the organization. Whether or not an organization's mission statement serves as an inspiration has more to do with how well and how consistently the people in the organization, particularly those who hold positions with the greatest power, act in ways that demonstrate their commitment to the organization's mission. Mission statements are often created at the higher echelons of organizations and may or may not reflect the beliefs and practices of those who work at the operational level.

Organizational Concepts and Models

Organizations are structured in a variety of ways.

- Vertical integration is an arrangement that provides different but complementary services among the parties involved; for example, the affiliation of a particular hospital with a health maintenance organization.
- Horizontal integration indicates shared or reciprocal services across two or more institutions; for example, the provision of cardiac surgical services by one affiliate and the provision of oncology services by the other.
- In a joint venture, one partner provides a needed service while the other partner assures financing for the service.
- Organizations or units within organizations may be structured by function or by product line. In a **functional** model, decision making is centralized and coordination among groups or entities may be lacking. A **matrix** structure integrates functions and products and by its very nature may "violate" the unity-of-command principle in that those who operate within this structure may have complex reporting relationships.

1

- **Shared governance** fosters ownership of the work to be done by formally involving those who perform it in decisions about structure, performance, staffing, and resource allocation.

Framework

The mission and vision of an organization are consistent with the organization's structural intent. For example, the mission statement for a small rural community hospital that provides a modest number of primary care services will reflect that reality, and its text will differ considerably from the mission statement of the huge academic tertiary center in a metropolitan area fifty miles away. The intent of both is to offer statements consistent with their particular aspirations, not to hold themselves out as something they are not.

The mission statements of academic health centers deserve brief, special mention. The reason many academic institutions devoted to health care exist is to provide a learning environment for practitioners in the early phase of their careers and to perform health-related research. The "caring language" characteristic of the mission statements of many community hospitals, even of those that are quite large or part of multi-hospital systems, may be missing from the mission statements of (some) academic institutions. Patient care may be listed as a secondary purpose.

Why is this distinction important? It is because those who seek employment in any organization should do their best to assure that their personal and professional values are in alignment with those of the institution before accepting a job offer.

Format

The mission and the vision statement are meant to instill confidence in those who seek care from the institution and pride in those who practice within its walls. They should be appealing in appearance, clear in their wording, understandable to the community at large, and easily recalled by the organization's staff.

Review Mechanisms

Mission and vision statements undergo periodic review to assure consistency with actual practice. In general, the mission, vision, and philosophy of an organization are carefully reviewed as part of the episodic accreditation process, whether through the Joint Commission on the Accreditation of Healthcare Organizations (JCAHO) or some other accrediting body.

THE PLANNING CONTINUUM

The planning process includes these steps: 1) assessment; 2) setting goals; 3) establishing objectives (plans); 4) determining actions. Planning addresses the *who, why, what, when, where, and how* an organization will function to achieve its intended objectives.

Strategic Planning

Strategic planning has to do with defining the long-term objectives of the organization and setting priorities. The timeline is future oriented and predicts organizational activities over a number of years. The capital building plan is an example of strategic planning.

Assessment

Assessment implies determining the strengths, weaknesses, opportunities, and threats (SWOT) that face the organization, analyzing risks, determining the preferred future state, and securing potential resources

Goal Setting

Strategic goals set the organization's path for several years into the future. To the extent the goals are consistent with the vision and values of the organization and are well defined, the greater the likelihood they will be achieved, absent unanticipated crises.

Prioritizing

Because there is always the possibility that a reversal of fortune could occur, organizations need to set priorities and get critical buy-ins from key stakeholders during the planning process. Dependencies need to be considered when establishing priorities in order to avoid unexpected surprises.

Evaluation

Measures of success need to be established at the outset so that the anticipated outcome of any strategic initiative is known in advance and can be measured on an ongoing basis.

1

Contingency Planning

Contingency planning has to do with managing the business in the moment and determining reactively or proactively what is to be done in the face of unexpected occurrences. In many ways contingency planning is the way businesses operate on a day-to-day basis.

Crisis Management

Crisis management has to do with the manner in which organizations respond to unexpected events over which they have little or no control. Since "uncontrollable" situations occur with relative frequency in health care, developing purposeful intervention strategies seems prudent.

Johnson & Johnson's handling of the Tylenol® crisis is often cited as an exemplary approach to crisis management and is consistent with the "truthful disclosure" approach health care organizations are beginning to take in order to maintain public trust. In 1982, seven people in the Chicago area died after taking Extra-Strength Tylenol® capsules that had been laced with cyanide. The containers had been tampered with after they left the manufacturing plant. Rather than claim that the company was not to blame, Johnson & Johnson (J&J) immediately launched a public relations program to preserve the integrity of the product and the company. Marketing experts believed that Tylenol® would disappear from pharmacy shelves never to be mentioned again, except in negative terms. However, J&J's leaders put public safety first and worried about financial impact later. They alerted consumers throughout the nation to avoid the consumption any Tylenol® product until the extent of the tampering could be determined. They stopped production of all Tylenol® products and recalled all Tylenol® capsules from the market at a cost of more than $100 million. They offered to replace any Tylenol® capsules people had already purchased with Tylenol® tablets. They quickly began working with the Chicago Police Department, the FBI, and the Federal Drug Administration (FDA). They put up $100,000 in reward money to help catch the perpetrator of the crime. Not only did the company survive and thrive, Tylenol® remains one of its biggest sellers and most profitable products. The forthright approach of the company reassured the community that its safety came first and that J&J cared enough to be publicly open and truthful about the crisis (Kaplan, 1998).

During the planning process, company leaders should ask and answer the followings questions as they prepare a crisis management intervention:

- What kind of crises could this company face?
- Does the organization have the capability to detect a crisis in its early stages?
- How will the organization manage a crisis if one occurs?
- How can the organization benefit from a crisis once it has passed?

1

With the answers to these questions in mind, the leadership can create a crisis management plan with these elements:

- Technical and structural actions — creating a crisis management team and allocating a budget for its functions.
- Evaluation and diagnostic actions — conducting various types of audits (e.g., threats and liabilities, environmental impact, and establishing a tracking system).
- Communication actions — communicating with the media, local communities, police, and government officials.
- Psychological and cultural actions — showing commitment to the crisis management plan early on.

Program Planning

Program planning takes into consideration the organization's capacity to successfully execute a particular plan or service. Programs selected by the organization must match the overall philosophy of the organization, be financially sound, and, in general, create a profit for the organization. Some programs may be mandated—for example, mental health services in a health maintenance environment—or voluntary, like a full-scope, freestanding women's health service.

STANDARDS

Standards are written statements that define expected performance. The following terms are used to describe types of standards: process, structure, and outcome. Structure standards pertain to the physical environment and management of an organization; process standards are those concerned with the actual delivery of care; outcome standards describe the intended result.

Here are examples of each:

- Structure (focus on institution or setting): The patient-care services division of HMS Medical Center operates under the direction of the Vice President for Nursing (VP-N). The VP-N is a member of the executive council.
- Process (focus on clinician, provider): Nurses practicing in the Oncology Service are certified in their specialty and practice according to the standards set forth by the Oncology Nursing Society.
- Outcome (focus on patient/client): Patients discharged from the intensive care unit to Level 2 care are physiologically stable, defined as (note parameters here).

1

Policies

Policies, procedures, protocols, and guidelines are tools that guide those who perform the work of the organization. Policy statements may be thought of as the "why" certain acts are performed or the conditions under which they are performed. For example, a policy statement might read: "Only registered nurses administer intravenous chemotherapy."

Procedures

Procedures describe in general terms how something is to be accomplished. Procedures answer the "what" and "how" questions. For example, "flush secondary line with normal saline before superimposing IV antibiotic."

Protocols

Protocols are more prescriptive and detail precise steps and their sequence for a given activity. For example, "prednisone rescue protocol for acute asthma flare: 20 mg bid x 3 days; 10 mg bid x 2 days, 5 mg bid x 2 days." Guidelines, on the other hand, describe the recommended approach for a given activity but still allow for discretion by the person performing the activity. For example: Consider adding HCTZ 12.5 to HTN control regimen if systolic BP remains > 145 after 1 month treatment with xxx." Guidelines, like protocols, should be evidence based.

Practice Standards

Standards are written statements that specify a level of performance or a set of conditions determined to be acceptable by a recognized authority. Standards are further defined as structure, process, and outcome.

Structure standards apply to the organizational environment, physical arrangements, and management. Process standards are concerned with the actual delivery of patient care. Outcome standards define the expected result of care provided.

Professional Criteria

The following standards of performance and practice, applicable to nursing administration, are derived from *Nursing Administration: Scope and Standards of Practice* (ANA, 2003). Amplification of the standards is found in the ANA monograph, a publication that is recommended to any nurse in a managerial or administrative role.

Standards of Practice

Standards of Practice are authoritative statements that describe a competent level of practice demonstrated through assessment, diagnosis/problem identification, identification of outcomes, planning, implementation, and evaluation.

- **Standard 1. Quality of Care and Administrative Practice**
  The nurse administrator systematically evaluates the quality and effectiveness of nursing practice and nursing services administration.

- **Standard 2. Diagnosis/Problem Identification**
  The nurse administrator develops, maintains, and evaluates an environment that empowers and supports the professional nurse in analysis of assessment data and in decisions to determine relevant diagnoses.

- **Standard 3. Identification of Outcomes**
  The nurse administrator develops, maintains, and evaluates information systems and processes that promote desired, client-defined, and organizational outcomes.

- **Standard 4. Planning**
  The nurse administrator develops, maintains, and evaluates organizational systems to facilitate planning for the delivery of nursing care.

- **Standard 5. Implementation**
  The nurse administrator develops, maintains, and evaluates organizational systems that support implementation of plans and delivery of care.

- **Standard 6. Evaluation**
  The nurse administrator evaluates the plan and its progress in relation to the attainment of outcomes.

Standards of Professional Performance

Standards of Professional Performance are authoritative statements that describe a competent level of behavior in the professional role, including activities related to quality of care and administrative practice, performance appraisal, education, professional environment, ethics, collaboration, research, and resource utilization.

- **Standard 1. Quality of Care and Administrative Practice**
  The nurse administrator systematically evaluates the quality and effectiveness of nursing practice and nursing services administration.

- **Standard 2. Performance Appraisal**
  The nurse administrator evaluates personal performance based on professional practice standards, relevant statutes and regulations, and organizational criteria.

- **Standard 3. Education**
  The nurse administrator maintains and demonstrates current knowledge in the administration of health care organizations to advance clinical practice.

1

- **Standard 4. Professional Environment**
  The nurse administrator is accountable for providing a professional environment.

- **Standard 5. Ethics**
  The nurse administrator's decisions and actions are based on ethical principles.

- **Standard 6. Collaboration**
  The nurse administrator collaborates with nursing staff at all levels, interdisciplinary teams, executive leaders, and other stakeholders.

- **Standard 7. Research**
  The nurse administrator supports research and its integration into nursing administration and the delivery of nursing care.

- **Standard 8. Resource Utilization**
  The nurse administrator evaluates and administers the resources of nursing services.

PRACTICE ENVIRONMENT

Nursing Care Delivery Systems/ Professional Practice Models

Here, briefly described, are several models of practice that have been embraced within the field of nursing over the years:

- Functional nursing — required tasks are divided among staff, with each nurse taking responsibility for executing an assigned function (e.g., "IV nurse," "dressing nurse," "procedure nurse"). This approach is not unlike the industrial model used in other segments of the business world.
- Team nursing — required care for a group of patients is carried out by several team members, such as the registered nurse, licensed practical nurse, nurse's aide and physical therapy aide. The RN serves in the role of team leader and as such has the opportunity to apply managerial skills as a means of accomplishing the work at hand.
- Primary nursing — the responsibility for the care of the patient, or group of patients, rests exclusively with the registered nurse. Primary nursing has been interpreted in a variety of ways: 1) the RN provides all care for the patient during her/his shift of duty; 2) the "primary" RN assumes 24-hour accountability for the care of the patient with "associates" overseeing the patient's care when the primary care RN is not in attendance; 3) while the nurse is the primary caregiver and cannot delegate authority, she/he is assisted by others in the provision of direct care while maintaining overall responsibility for the patient. The core

elements of primary nursing include: continuity of care for the patient; account-ability of the nurse for the patient's care; care that is comprehensive, individual-ized, and coordinated; and the professional satisfaction of the nurse.

■ Total patient care — this mode of practice is akin to the first approach described above under primary nursing. The registered nurse cares exclusively for one or a small group of patients. This mode of practice is common in specialty services such as intensive care.

Governance Models

As with governance higher in the organizational structure, unit level governance can take a variety of forms. In a traditional hierarchy, lead staff report to a charge nurse, who in turn reports to a nurse manager, who then reports to a unit manager/coor-dinator or assistant manager and so on up the chain of command.

A newer model, that of shared governance, suggests that this approach to unit management may be more successful in the long run. Shared governance allows staff nurses to be part of the decision-making process about the organization of work on their unit or service. For example, the 22 entities that make up the Seton Healthcare Network in Central Texas embrace shared governance. Seton has established a Nursing Practice Congress, which meets monthly to "collectively set and evaluate nursing care standards across the Network." According to Seton's public relation's materials, "Shared governance empowers frontline staff nurses to actively partici-pate on policy-making bodies that determine the professional nursing practice envi-ronment at SETON. The integrity of the governance model relies upon meaningful participation of staff nurses—at meetings of staff, department Practice Councils, Specialty Councils, and the Nursing Congress." Several of the network's facilities have been awarded ANCC Magnet Recognition status.

The assumed outcome in the presence of shared governance is greater accounta-bility for practice, greater staff satisfaction, improved clinical outcomes, and greater efficiency. Labor-management partnerships in unionized environments strive for similar outcomes.

Differential Practice

In this model, the care delivered is based on the educational level and expertise of the nurses who assume responsibility for one or more patients. For example, a clin-ical nurse specialist, a registered nurse, and a licensed practical nurse may each con-tribute to the patient's care and collaborate in such a way that each brings her/his particular skills to bear in assuring that the patient receives needed care. In another sense, differentiated nursing care defines specialization (e.g., renal nursing, burn unit nursing, ambulatory care nursing, etc.).

In differentiated nursing care/case management, the registered nurse is placed in the position of effectively managing the care of a group of patients as they move

1

through the continuum of care, perhaps from the inpatient setting, to the convalescent setting, to the home with the assistance of home care, and eventually to independence. Case management is a growing field for nurses in all settings.

Case Management

Case managers coordinate needed care for a designated group of patients based on defined characteristics of the group. Third-party payers may employ case managers. Case managers are responsible for reviewing the cost and relative effectiveness of proposed care and recommend approval or denial of the requested intervention. They may also suggest alternative, less costly interventions. Registered nurses constitute the largest group of case managers employed by insurance providers and work closely with the medical directors of these same plans.

Case or care managers also practice in health care organizations where they coordinate care for various groups of patients, often by disease category (e.g., diabetes, asthma, heart failure). Case/care management is a growing field within nursing and is generally seen as a satisfying career choice.

Good research models for determining the effectiveness of case/care management are being developed and applied in the field. Despite empirical claims that the programs are effective, how effective they are is yet to be determined. Because of the nature of the population served, "true" cost savings may not be achieved, at least longitudinally. This possibility needs to be balanced against the probability that case management is the "right thing" to do, whether or not it significantly reduces costs.

Critical and Clinical Pathways

Clinical pathways define intended outcomes and provide direction for care. They are variously known as clinical practice guidelines, protocols, critical paths, and so forth. They may apply to care provided in one setting (e.g., the hospital), or they may extend across the continuum of care. They are generally developed and intended for use by multidisciplinary teams and are evidence based (the recommended actions are based on scientific studies to the extent such studies have been done). As with other such instruments, they follow the "law of averages" and variation must be explained or justified. Clinical pathways may be prescriptive ("do it this way") or descriptive ("this is the recommendation").

The extent to which clinical pathways form the foundation for practice is as yet unknown. Even though such guidelines exist in all care settings, the degree of buy-in on the part of the various disciplines has not reached critical mass. Nonetheless, as regulatory agencies and quality oversight groups look more closely at variation in practice, the likelihood that clinical pathways will be implemented and followed increases.

While it may be a matter of semantics, the concept of "critical path," as opposed to "clinical path," may benefit by clarification. The term "critical path" is actually derived from the profit management literature. The critical path is set up in such a way that target timelines for critical elements are established. In addition, the steps along the path are sequential, with the beginning of the next step contingent on successful completion of the prior step. Software programs for critical path management are available.

Alternative Care Settings

The variety of settings in which nurses practice is broad and ever expanding. Here are just a few of the options available to nurses whose practice extends beyond the hospital.

- Ambulatory care
- Rehabilitation centers
- Schools and student health services
- Industrial and corporate nursing
- Long-term care
- Armed services
- Public health
- Research
- Nurse-managed community clinics
- Case management or utilization management within a managed care organization
- Parish nursing

Nurses have increasing opportunities to demonstrate their value in settings beyond the hospital. The extent to which nurses are perceived as contributors to the success of any endeavor, the better the public may come to understand the significant contribution that nurses make to the field of health care.

Corporate Culture and Climate

Corporate culture is characterized by a system of shared actions, values, and beliefs that develops within an organization and guides the behavior of its members. Corporate culture is a pervasive force and its power is not always appreciated unless it is breached either intentionally or unintentionally.

Culture helps those within the organization define the characteristics of their organization, helps those new to the organization to "fit in," and clarifies the organization to those outside its boundaries. Awareness of the organization's culture in advance of employment helps potential employees determine if their own values and those of the organization are in synergy. If they are not, then the applicant may elect to seek employment with another company. Corporate culture can change, but it rarely does so in response to a single individual.

Those who observe such phenomena believe that cultural differences have a major impact on the performance of organizations and the quality of work life experienced by those within the organization.

1

Autocratic

The autocratic organization is generally perceived as a "top down" entity with decisions made at the executive level, then announced to the workforce. Managers and administrators are expected to enforce the decisions, thus their efforts are directed toward helping staff accept decisions that have already been made. Techniques used to gain compliance include coercion, threats of punishment, and clear direction of actions.

While autocracy certainly has its detractors—and it is hardly a preferred practice in today's business environment—there may be times when an autocratic approach means the difference between success and failure of a business, particularly a business that finds itself in crisis with a very short window of opportunity for turnaround.

Bureaucratic

A bureaucratic culture is characterized by reliance on rules, regulations, policies, and procedures. While all organizations need practical policies and procedures in order to avoid chaos, rules are central to the bureaucratic organization. Proponents of the bureaucratic approach believe that personnel compliance with the norms of the organization can best be achieved through external motivation engendered by fear of reprisal if rules are broken. Some tout government agencies as the classical example of bureaucracy, even labeling staff members as "bureaucrats." In reality, many bureaucratic organizations, health care institutions among them, exist outside of government, and a good many government agencies now operate in a participative manner.

Participative

A participative culture is characterized by openness to input from all levels within the organization as part of the decision-making process. It is important to distinguish input from the actual decisions leaders must make. Employees are sometimes disappointed when the final decision is contrary to or significantly different from the suggestions they have given. In a participative culture, managers and administrators have an obligation to let employees know in advance how their input will be used.

Those who subscribe to a participative philosophy believe that employees are internally motivated to achieve the goals of the organization because their personal values are consistent with those of the organization. Employees respond more favorably to encouragement and coaching than to top-down direction, to rule-bound dictates, or to reprimand.

The term *situational* is sometimes used to describe the leadership style that may be seen in a participative culture. Here is a "shorthand" version of the continuum of options available to the manager:

- Decide — manager makes decision, may or may not get input from individuals or groups prior to announcing the decision;
- Consult individually — problem presented to group members individually, input obtained, manager decides;

- Consult group — problem presented to group as a whole, input obtained, manager decides;
- Facilitate — problem presented to group, boundaries set by manager, manager facilitates group but has no greater say in outcome than any other member of the group, group decides;
- Delegate — manager sets boundaries for the group then steps out of active participation in the work of the group, provides behind-the-scenes resources and encouragement, group decides.

Collaborative Practice

Collaborative practice takes place when members of various disciplines, each with a particular set of skills needed by the patient/family, come together to plan and deliver care. The American Nurses Association describes collaboration as a partnership in which power on both sides is valued, recognized, and accepted. The term initially came into use as intentional collaboration between the disciplines of nursing and medicine was being formalized.

Career Ladder

Clinical ladders foster recognition of clinically expert nurses and offer a career pathway that allows them to continue providing direct care to patients. In general, those who elect to "climb" the clinical ladder need to demonstrate their expertise through testimony of colleagues and supervisors and presentation of exemplars clearly detailing how their application of the nursing process has made a difference in the outcome of care for one or more clients/patients. This process has been well outlined by Patricia Benner and her colleagues in the classic text From Novice to Expert (Benner, 1984).

The career ladder may be seen somewhat differently; it suggests that the nurse will move intentionally through a career path that builds on and fosters development of her/his leadership skills—perhaps moving "through the ranks" from charge nurse to manager and eventually to an executive-level position— depending on skill, education, and the availability of sponsorship and mentoring.

Consistent with ANA's standards of performance and practice for nursing administrators, those who desire to move into the administrative rank of nursing have an obligation to prepare themselves to do so both academically and experientially.

Alternatively, the nurse's career ladder may take a more clinical direction, moving from staff nurse to clinical nurse specialist or perhaps to nurse practitioner or educator.

Collaboration and Consultation

The American Nurses Association describes collaboration as a partnership in which power on both sides is valued, recognized, and accepted. Collaboration implies that various parties, physicians and nurses in particular, engage in joint problem solving with the best interest of the client(s) foremost in mind. The parties are characterized as having "separate and combined spheres of activity and responsibility, mutual safeguarding of legitimate interests of each party," and common goals. In a management sense, collaboration means that the involved parties come together to solve the problem in an atmosphere of mutual respect. This approach is of particular value when the goals of both parties are too critical to be compromised.

Consultation occurs when the knowledge needed to better identify a problem rests outside the staff member's current realm or scope of practice. The consultant brings her/his expertise and objectivity to the problem-solving process. The person requesting the consultation recognizes her/his own limitations, gains valuable insight during the consultation process, and is then able to apply these learnings in other situations. For example, the new nurse manager may request consultation with the corporate controller or with the financial analyst to better understand the budget process. In the clinical setting, the nurse new to the oncology clinic may request consultation with the highly experienced clinical nurse specialist in establishing a care plan for the patient with acute myelogenous leukemia undergoing experimental chemotherapy.

Integrated Health Care System (e,g., networks, consortia)

In an integrated system, providers agree to accept the risk of caring for a particular segment of the population for a pre-established fee and to provide needed care across the continuum in a cost-effective manner. Preventive care is inherent in this system, with primary care providers, not the hospital, at the center of the equation. Keeping people healthy is seen as a way to use resources most efficiently; therefore, decreasing the need for hospitalization is both goal and outcome of the integrated health care system.

Systems may be vertically or virtually integrated. In vertical integration, hospitals, medical groups, and other delivery system elements are brought together under one umbrella. There is a shared purpose and unity of control. Virtually integrated systems are those that are linked contractually; purpose is shared, but control remains more or less autonomous. Potential challenges in vertical integration include relatively high overhead and internal power struggles. On the other hand, the virtually integrated groups may remain committed to being a part of the system only to extent that the new system is perceived as more advantageous than any other alternative.

For health care organizations that have their own "brand identity" to form a consortium with other organizations, the culture of each organization should be thoroughly assessed for compatibility. To leave relationships to chance or to automatically assume that greater integration will occur because of a pronouncement can prove to be a disaster.

INSTITUTIONAL ENVIRONMENT

Organizational Structure

Centralized versus Decentralized

The centralized organization is a typical hierarchy that follows the traditional chain-of-command concept. It is characterized by top-down decision making. The more decision making is "pushed down" the chain of command, the more decentralized the organization becomes. With increased decentralization, lower level managers have more opportunity to develop their executive skills and achieve greater job satisfaction.

Product Line

Product line structure, structure by specialization, has several advantages: task assignments are clear and are related to employees' skills; employees can build on one another's knowledge, training, and experience; new managers have a ready-made laboratory in which to enhance their skills; and the product line is easy to explain.

Product lines can be further characterized as functional or divisional. The term functional is self-explanatory. For example, surgical oncology, head injury rehabilitation, and endocrinology can be characterized as functional product lines. Divisional product lines cluster products, services, clients, and/or legal entities in geographically dispersed areas with the intent of increasing market share. Critics of divisional dispersion suggest that duplication of effort and service may occur under this model and thus the hypothetical advantages of the product line may be compromised.

Matrix

Matrix organizations combine functional and divisional patterns and assign individuals to more than one unit. From the perspective of classic managerial theory, the matrix model defies the unity-of-command principle in that it requires employees to report to more than one "boss." In practical terms, and with the complexity of the modern workplace, the matrix organization makes sense and may occur "organically"— that is, it will simply come into being because it works; or "purposely"—that is, it will be intentionally created because of its value.

Exquisite communication is required for a matrix organization to succeed. In the absence of open, dynamic formal and informal communication links, the overlapping authority and responsibility of managers may lead to conflicts, gaps in productivity, and inconsistent practice.

Committee Structure

A committee brings together a group of people with the intent of achieving a common task or goal. Committees may be formal or informal; they may be permanent or ad hoc (convened for a short time for a particular purpose). An ad hoc committee

1

may be termed a task force. The existence of certain committees is specified in the organization's bylaws and may be mandated by external regulatory agencies.

To the extent possible, committee size should be such that work can be accomplished consistent with principles of group formation and cohesiveness. Groups of five to ten tend to accomplish their assigned tasks more efficiently than larger groups. If the committee must be large in order to meet political or organizational intent, then the creation of subcommittees within the group may help the committee move its work forward more quickly.

Planning is key to committee success. In an ideal situation:

- The agenda should be well planned and published in advance.
- The committee should ideally create a charter for itself so that its intent and link to the larger organization is clear.
- Each meeting should have a stated purpose.
- Participants should come to the committee with their assignments complete and ready to participate fully in the work of the group.
- Opposing viewpoints should be welcomed and respected.
- The group should remain focused.
- Ground rules should be established early on.
- Meaningful reports should be generated as a result of the committee's work.
- Time spent in committee meetings and in the accomplishment of committee tasks should further the goals of the organization.
- Meetings should start and end on time.

Governing Boards

The board of directors of an organization makes major decisions affecting the organization. The board is led by a chairperson, governed by a set of bylaws, and is responsible for discharging the following duties: 1) selecting, assessing, rewarding, and sometimes replacing the chief executive officer (CEO); 2) determining the strategic direction of the organization and reviewing its financial performance; 3) assuring that the activities of the organization are ethical, socially responsible, and legal.

Systems Integration

Networks

Networks allow entities to come together as a way of providing greater value to a community, as a means to consolidate power or market share, or as a mode to enhance fiscal solvency through collective purchasing power.

Network relationships allow for organizational autonomy on one hand and coalitional power on the other. For example, several hospitals in a particular geographical area may determine that it is in their best interest to form a coalition for the purpose of joint purchasing and contracting. However, each of the facilities retains its independent internal system of governance.

1

The concept of network also applies to communications. Communication networks may be decentralized, centralized, or restricted. In a decentralized system, direct communication occurs up, down, across, in, and out without restriction. Centralized communication implies that input and output is controlled to a greater or lesser extent through a "hub" or control point. Restricted networks place intentional barriers between groups, particularly those that disagree with one another's positions.

Management Information Systems

Management information systems (MIS) are essential to the business of health care. MIS represents an almost staggering investment of resources in order to assure that the systems needed to conduct business, document clinical care, capture trends, and meet the demands of regulatory bodies and purchasers are in place. The rapidity with which technology is changing means not only an initial investment, but also ongoing capital and operational expenditures.

Organizations related to health care management information systems have come into existence in recent years, as have careers in the area of MIS. Medical records administrators and clinical librarians are but two of the careers that have changed dramatically with the advent of MIS. Indeed, these job titles themselves are nearly obsolete. It is not uncommon to see a chief information officer (CIO) integrated into the executive level of the organizational chart of health care organizations.

A few short years ago, the acronyms "WAN" (wide area network) and "LAN" (local area network) were alien terms to the majority of administrators and clinicians alike. Now an entire vocabulary of technology terms sits alongside the medical lexicon.

The term local area network (LAN) refers to a number of personal computers linked together through a "server." The concept is somewhat akin to an office that has several phone lines, each connected to the other, though able to be used independently.

Wide area networks are made up of local area networks, and the system can be enlarged exponentially. Connections are effected by specialized networking software and are transparent to the user.

Nursing has its own association, the American Nursing Informatics Association (ANIA), whose members are involved with or interested in the field of nursing informatics. The American Nurses Association describes nursing informatics as the integration of "nursing science, computer science and information science to manage and communicate data, information and knowledge in nursing practice."

Electronic data transfer fosters the integration of care across the continuum. However, the promise of the fully functional computerized medical record is yet to be realized. As those who practice in the field of informatics have learned, the complexity of health care is such that the anticipated migration from paper to "bits and bytes" has yet to occur on a large scale. Nonetheless, the **electronic health record** will eventually become a near-universal reality. An understanding of semantics related to the computerization of medical and health records is useful. The **automated medical record** (AMR) is considered a "first-level" product that brings together information from other sources. The record is delivered electronically to an end user for his/her use in caring for the patient. However, the end user cannot immediately enter data (respond to) what s/he has received (i.e., the AMR is not interactive). The next level is termed the **computerized medical record system,** in which paper-based products now become available electronically through scanning. The **electronic medical record** is the third-level product; it provides capability for electronic data entry, electronic signature, data integrity, and audit tools. The **electronic patient record** is the fourth-level product; it brings together information about the patient from more than one organization, thus supporting the argument for a universally agreed upon "e-language" and code. Finally, **electronic health record** is the fifth-level product, including information about the person's well-being from multiple sources, not only about her/his medical problems.

The Internet

The "World Wide Web" or the "electronic highway" represents a phenomenon without parallel. The instantaneous availability of information and the ability to connect with the person next door or colleagues half a world away does indeed make planet Earth seem a bit smaller.

The Internet is changing the way medicine—and by extension, nursing—is practiced. Patients are engaged in self-care as never before. They approach their providers with the latest articles about illness, medications, treatments, and research in hand, hot off the printer! Expectations have changed; relationships have been altered. While the concept of "patient as partner" or "patient as leader of her/his health team" is not yet a universally embraced concept, it is clearly on the horizon.

Telehealth is no longer in the realm of science fiction. Nurses using laptops and small video cameras videotape the patient in her/his residence in real time. The recording can be transmitted immediately to other health care providers so that assessment and needed intervention can occur in the moment. The transmission is not constrained by time or distance; thus, patients in remote locations can enjoy the same level of consultation as those who live adjacent to medical centers. Radiologists read digitized images from a location far removed from the diagnostic imaging department. Laboratory data are transmitted via secure servers from location to location. There are few barriers in the virtual world save for the electronic security "firewalls" purposely incorporated into information systems. Many organizations take advantage of the firewall concept to create intranet systems that allow communication only within defined boundaries. The Office for the Advancement of Telehealth (OAT) now exists as a division within the Health Resources and Services Administration (HRSA), itself a division of the Department of Health and Human Services (HHS) (**www.hrsa.gov/telehealth**).

As with any seemingly wondrous invention, the Internet also brings with it a cautionary tale. The accuracy and source of information must be carefully scrutinized. It is incumbent upon health care professionals to assist patients and families in distinguishing information that is of high quality from that which is questionable or even harmful. Vigilance is also called for with regard to "hackers" who "break into" systems, sometimes with the intent to harm, at other times simply for the thrill of proving they can "scale the wall."

Continuity of Care

Continuity of care implies that the services needed to promote the patient's/client's health and well-being are coordinated within and across the continuum of services provided in the outpatient, inpatient, rehabilitative, or continuing care setting and home care/hospice. At each point in the process, the patient's/family's preferences and values should be taken into consideration along with the needs and demands of the organization.

In the acute or extended care settings, discharge planners, generally nurses or social workers, play a key role in assuring that the needs of the patient are anticipated at the next level of care to which s/he proceeds.

Well-orchestrated continuity of care assures that the needs of the patient are met in the most cost-effective manner possible. This ideal is often frustrated because of the fragmentation that characterizes the current health system.

Restructuring

Organizations restructure in response to a variety of internal or external factors. Restructuring is seen as a means to reduce duplication of effort and to increase productivity. A caveat: The investment in restructuring to gain promised efficiencies needs to be examined carefully. Such scrutiny should occur before the initiation of restructuring efforts. However, the dubious investment in restructuring is sometimes identified only after the fact.

Internal

Internal restructuring refers to a change in communication channels, reporting relationships, the function of various business units or departments within an organization, or even to the restructuring of job titles and duties.

External

External restructuring follows the decision to integrate disparate entities or in the presence of mergers or new affiliations. For example, two hospitals in close proximity to one another may elect to merge their establishments (provided, of course, they meet any legal challenges encountered along the way). As a result of the merger, only one administrative team is needed, and this is generally a combination of the two previously existing teams. Severance packages may be offered to those whose positions are now redundant or they may be offered other positions within the new organization.

1

EXTERNAL ENVIRONMENT

The health care system is not confined to hospitals or clinics. Rather, it is composed of a far-reaching network of affiliates, regulatory agencies, and special interest groups or organizations.

Community Organizations

Community organizations exist to serve the needs of defined populations or to promote and garner resources for specific activities. Community clinics are often established to serve the needs of those with low incomes and/or the uninsured. Government funding through defined allocations or grants, supplemented by private contributions, often through foundations, constitutes the funding source for community clinics. For example, in 1999 the Tides Foundation established the Community Clinics Initiative (CCI) in the state of California in order to improve the technology and information systems of California's nonprofit community clinics.

The American Red Cross, the American or Canadian Lung Associations, the Muscular Dystrophy Society, the American Diabetes Association, and the American Heart Association are but a few of the many examples of community organizations, many funded largely with donations from private citizens, that exist to provide a variety of services to those in need.

Access to Care

Access to care may be defined as the entry into or use of health care services. Access is generally seen as inseparable from cost and quality; that is, cost, quality, and access are generally addressed as the balancing forces that lead to improvement or disintegration of health, whether of an individual or of a community. Paradoxically, increased access may in some cases actually decrease the cost of care, or lessened expenditures may improve the quality of care. For example, the person with diabetes who has access to early intervention and ongoing support through the health care system supplemented with involvement in the local Diabetes Society may stay in better control of her diabetes and avoid the devastating and costly cardiovascular and renal sequelae of diabetes.

The dimensions of access include:

- Geographical access is impacted by where people live in relation to where services are available. Someone living in a remote area of Alaska will not have the same geographic access to care as a person living in metropolitan Chicago.
- Physical access is influenced by the capability and mobility of people to reach the locations where care is provided.

- Temporal access refers to the match between the hours the health care system is available and the relative convenience of those hours to people who seek care.
- Sociocultural access refers to the match between expectations of a given cultural group and the ability of the health care system to meet those expectations.
- Financial access to care is mediated by the ability to pay for services provided. In the United States, most financial access to care is through third-party payers (i.e., insurance of one type or another).

Community Assessment, Demographic Assessment, and Feasibility Studies

Studies are conducted in order to determine priority health needs and the gaps in services and systems required to meet those needs in a defined geographical location. Such studies measure the prevalence of chronic health conditions, the need and adequacy of mental health and substance abuse services, demographics, socioeconomic trends, the need for and adequacy of acute care, long-term care, specialty care, public health services, and so forth. Findings then become the stimulus for new initiatives and for community and/or professional education. Whether the studies are undertaken locally as a discreet task or by one of the many public policy institutes available for such activities depends on the scope, intent, and funding allocated for the study.

Community Diagnosis and Epidemiology

Epidemiology refers to the study of the prevalence of a disease or health condition and the factors that determine its prevalence. Protection of the public is implied and, as such, epidemiology is concerned with the health of populations rather than of individuals. Descriptive epidemiology takes into consideration time, place, and person. Analytic epidemiology is concerned with the agent, host, and environment, and, as a matter of course, follows descriptive epidemiology.

Interagency Relationships

Various agencies involved with the delivery of health care form or are obligated to maintain relationships with one another. For example, hospitals are obligated to inform the Public Health Department about the occurrence of certain infectious diseases; the Centers for Medicare and Medicaid Services (CMS), formerly the Health Care Financing Administration (HCFA), is obligated to inform care delivery systems of changes in reimbursement policies for care provided to Medicare and Medicaid recipients.

In a wholly integrated system—which the U.S. health care system is not—such relationships would likely be better defined that they are at present.

1

Health Care Industry

The term "health care industry" refers to the conglomerate of products, people, and services involved with the delivery of health care in the United States. Make no mistake, health care is "big business"—it is a trillion dollar industry! As of the year 2000, the Gross Domestic Product (GDP) devoted to health care-related expenditures was 13.2%, up from 8.8% in 1980. Analysts predict that the percent of financial resources devoted to health care will continue to grow in the years ahead.

Driving forces include drugs, medical devices and other medical advances (22%); general inflation (18%); rising provider expenses (18%); government mandates and regulations (15%); increased consumer demand (15%); litigation and risk management (7%); and other factors (5%).

Total spending by private health insurance is expected to increase from $537 billion in 2002 to $767 billion in 2007, an annual growth rate of 7.4% (Price, Waterhouse, Coopers, April 2002). This figure assumes a continuation of some cost restraint provided by managed care. In the absence of managed care, the analytical model predicts a figure of $833 billion in 2007.

National and International Factors

While the United States spends more pre capita on health care than any other industrialized nation, the health care expenditures in other developed countries are also rising regardless of the system of care in place in those countries. The rise in cost is fueled by factors similar to those identified above and in particular the changing demographics that show a significant rise in the number of elderly persons. The extent to which costs can be contained in the near term remains in question. Other sectors of the economy compete for the same resources and may lay claim to the possibility that a shift in expenditures away from the health care industry toward other sectors may actually do more to improve the overall health of a nation. For example, greater access to education is linked to better health. Relatively inexpensive public health interventions decrease the spread of communicable disease and improve the health of those with limited resources. Personal choice and lifestyle modifications significantly decrease the incidence of chronic disease. On a global level, the need to care for people with AIDS and to decrease the incidence of AIDS remains a very real challenge

Health Care Policy

Health care policy is established largely through government agencies, chief among them the U.S. Department of Health and Human Services at the national level and department equivalents at the state level.

The following initiatives are among the most significant for the development of broad-based health policy in the current and coming decades.

1

Healthy People 2010: Understanding and Improving Health

Published under the auspices of the U.S. Public Health Service, this text builds on the seminal document first issued in 1991 and on *Healthy People 2000: National Health Promotion and Disease Prevention Objectives* (**www.healthypeople.gov**).

Healthy People 2010 is the prevention agenda for the nation. It is a statement of national health objectives designed to identify the most significant preventable threats to health and to establish national goals to reduce these threats.

Healthy People is managed by the Office of Disease Prevention and Health Promotion, U.S. Department of Health and Human Services. It has two main goals:

- **Goal 1:** Increase Quality and Years of Healthy Life. The first goal of Healthy People 2010 is to help individuals of all ages increase life expectancy and improve their quality of life.

- **Goal 2:** Eliminate Health Disparities. The second goal of Healthy People 2010 is to eliminate health disparities among different segments of the population.

Guidelines of the U.S. Public Health Service's Centers
for Disease Control and Prevention

The recommended prevention guidelines, designed to keep people healthy, are used as a reference point for health promotion by a multitude of health plans throughout the United States.

Clinical Practice Guidelines for the U.S. Public Health Service's Agency
for Healthcare Research and Quality (AHRQ) (formerly the Agency for
Health Care Policy and Research)

Numerous evidence-based guidelines for practice, written from both the client's and the provider's perspectives, are available through AHRQ.

PHYSICAL ENVIRONMENT

Structural Design and Renovation

The physical environment in which health care services are provided is seen as important to the healing process. Patients and their families voice approval or disapproval of their surroundings and relate the comfort of the care setting to the overall quality of care provided. Health care design has become its own sub-specialty within the health care industry.

Design specialists are working in particular on the creation of safe, attractive environments in the area of long-term care; most notably, Alzheimer and dementia care facilities. Wellness communities and models such as Planetree, which has as part of its mission "to cultivate the healing of mind, body and spirit," are having an influence on the more mainstream sector of the health care design business. The purposeful use of color, texture, light, and sound contribute to a sense of well-being on the part of the patient as well as that of the staff.

Health care settings designed with the functions of the staff in mind contribute to employee efficiency and to a decrease in illness or injury on the part of the staff.

Participant Roles

The list of those involved in the design of the physical environment in which health care takes place is virtually endless. Frontline staff and managers as well as project managers, architects, design engineers, construction engineers, safety and regulatory experts, physicians and other clinicians, executive level decision makers, financial analysts, and others are called upon to participate in some way in the design process.

It is important that those who participate in various aspects of the design process are clear about their roles. For most managers and frontline staff, the role is consultative, not decision-making. The input of frontline personnel is essential in that they are most familiar with day-to-day workflow. On the other hand, the expertise of architects and design engineers is needed to create a functional space in compliance with the countless regulatory mandates in which the care will take place.

Occupancy Approval

Before patients can occupy any bed in any health care facility, approval for occupancy must be granted. Generally, occupancy approval is part of the licensing process and it rests with the state, though local surrogates, for example, a designated local fire chief, may participate in the preliminary and final review process.

Architectural Review

The regulatory requirements for health care institution construction or remodeling are among the most stringent in existence. Not only must the initial plan undergo scrutiny at numerous levels, but every change, even the smallest adjustment, must undergo review and be approved in advance of construction. Adjustments that occur after construction begins are similarly subject to close review and approval.

Safety and Code Requirements

Federal and state agencies govern the safety of the environments in which care is provided. The Occupational Safety and Health Administration is the predominant federal agency concerned with the codes that pertain to health care environments. Each state has a parallel agency that is established for like reasons but is customized to the needs of a particular state. For example, a state known to experience earthquakes is likely to have a stricter code of seismic safety than a state in which earthquakes do not pose a threat.

Because of its purpose, clientele, and relative risk for harm to clients should safety codes be breached, health care safety codes are extremely rigorous. Organizations must have systems and processes in place to assure compliance with all code requirements and must test their systems on an ongoing basis.

Efficiency

Environmental design should contribute to the efficiency of practice in a given unit. On one hand, the unit should be designed to accommodate the needs of the patients that will be housed there and the staff who will practice on the unit. On the other hand, given the dynamic nature of health care, a unit designed exclusively with today's patient population in mind may be obsolete before the doors open.

Still, a few principles are relatively universal and constant over time:

- Staff should be able to visualize as many patients as possible from their assigned workstation.
- Patients should be provided with privacy and quiet; family needs should be taken into consideration.
- There should be sufficient storage space to assure that the appearance of the unit is not cluttered.
- Workstations should meet stringent ergonomic standards, including proper lighting.
- The work unit should conserve energy for the staff; for example, if long halls are necessary because of design constraints, workstations should be decentralized.

Effects on Patients/Clients and Staff

None other than Florence Nightingale identified the positive effects of a pleasing environment on health, healing, and well being! Ancient practitioners, too, identified the importance of creating pleasant surroundings as part of the art of healing.

Research into the design and furnishing of long-term care facilities is an especially robust field at the moment. Whenever possible, clients or potential clients are involved in the design process.

The intentional use of color, artwork, lighting, and sound create an atmosphere that can contribute to the well-being of staff and patients.

1

PROGRAM EVALUATION

Program Evaluation Models

Various modes of program evaluation exist within the field of healthcare. The Joint Commission on Accreditation of Healthcare Organizations (JCAHO) is referenced at greater length in another section of this study guide. JCAHO has long been regarded as the standard-bearer with regard to the evaluation first of acute care facilities and more recently long-term, specialty and ambulatory care entities. JCAHO standards incorporate structure, process and outcome evaluation.

The National Committee for Quality Assurance focuses on quality measures that show the degree of improvement in clinical practice, with a focus on evidence-based interventions. The 2002 NCQA report, *The State of Health Care Quality 2002: Industry Trends and Analysis* revealed that the quality of health care is improving, but also cautioned that there is still room for improvement. By its own calculations, NCQA estimated that more than 6000 deaths and 22 million sick days could be avoided annually if identified "best practices" were more widely adopted.

NCQA's Health Plan Employer Data and Information Set (HEDIS) measures are used by employer groups and benefits managers to determine the comparative quality of a particular health plans and health systems and to make recommendations to employees about their choice of health plan during the open enrollment period.

The National Database of Nursing Quality Indicators (NDNQI) is linked with the American Nurses Association Quality and Safety Initiative. Systematic data collection from more than 250 hospitals throughout the United States helps researchers determine how, if, and/or to what degree nursing impacts patient outcomes. In addition to collecting patient care data, NDNQI also conducts a survey of nurse satisfaction (**www.nursingquality.org**).

The National Forum for Healthcare Quality Measurement and Reporting (NQF), incorporated in 1999, is a not-for-profit, public-private collaborative created to develop and implement a national strategy for health care quality measurement and reporting. NQF's member groups work to promote a common approach to measuring health care quality and fostering system-wide capacity for quality improvement. The organization came into being because of a "shared sense of urgency about the impact of health care quality on patient outcomes, workforce productivity, and health care costs," and the need to "bring about national change" (**www.qualityforum.org**).

Performance Improvement (PI)/Continuous Quality Improvement (CQI)/Total Quality Management (TQM)

Performance improvement (PI) activities are now firmly embedded in the quality structure of most organizations, particularly those that seek JCAHO accreditation. The plan-do-check-act (PDCA) cycle provides a model that is relatively easy to understand and that is able to graphically represent change over time with the use of tools such as control charts. It provides a common language and a wide variety of tools to help all personnel engaged in the process.

The philosophy underlying continuous quality improvement (CQI) is to continually raise the quality bar. As a particular goal is achieved and improvement sustained, the stakes are raised for the same goal. For example, if the baseline statistic for documentation of patient teaching consistent with the policies of the organization is 90%, and the long-term goal is 95%, perhaps the interim goal is 92%, followed the next year by 94%, and, finally, in the third year, if change is sustained, the bar is raised to 95%. Measurement continues until tools, techniques, and behavior patterns are part of daily practice for a period of months or years. Those involved with the project must then determine if the bar can be raised still higher, say to 98%, or if 95% is acceptable. In the latter situation, the staff would move on to another performance improvement initiative.

The CQI process helps organizations focus on the "vital few" interventions that are likely to have the most applicability to health outcomes and/or to continued accreditation.

In organizations that embrace total quality management (TQM), everyone is committed to continuous improvement in her/his part of the organization. The principles of TQM were articulated by W. Edwards Deming and Joseph Juran, both of whom worked in post-World War II Japan to help restart that country's industries in the wake of war's devastation. As some would say, "the rest is history," in that the impact of TQM on Japan's post-conflict economy was astounding. (The current world economy in developed countries does not reveal the "rosy" picture of a decade ago; a recessionary environment, including devaluation of the stock market, is taking its toll. Still, TQM's impact on productivity and quality is well documented.)

Deming's holistic approach maintains that the interaction of materials, machines, and people determines productivity, quality, and competitive advantage. Deming's 14 points further articulate the foundation of TQM:

- Create constancy of purpose; strive for long-term improvements rather than short-term profit.
- Adopt the new philosophy; do not tolerate delays and mistakes.
- Cease dependence on mass inspection; build quality into the process on the front end.
- End the practice of awarding business on price tag alone; build long-term relationships.
- Improve constantly and forever the system of production and service at each stage.
- Institute training and retraining; continually update methods and thinking.
- Institute leadership; provide resources needed for effectiveness.
- Drive out fear; people must believe it is safe to report problems or to ask for help.
- Break down barriers between departments; promote teamwork.
- Eliminate slogans, exhortations, and arbitrary targets; supply methods, not buzzwords.
- Eliminate numerical quotas; they are contrary to the idea of continuous improvement.

- Remove barriers to pride in workmanship; allow autonomy and spontaneity.
- Institute a vigorous program of education and retraining; people are assets, not commodities.
- Take action to accomplish the transformation; provide a structure that enables quality (Deming, 2000).

The Malcolm Baldrige Quality Award was created to honor businesses that best exemplify commitment to TQM. The application process is intense and rigorous. In general, the businesses that originally competed for the Baldrige Award were industrial manufacturing or service organizations. More recently, health care-specific criteria were established. In 2002 the St. Louis-based SSM Health Care Organization became the first health care organization to win the coveted Baldrige Award for its exceptional service and achievements in the area of quality improvement.

ANCC's Magnet Recognition Program also honors health care facilities and systems that "demonstrate sustained excellence in nursing care." As of 2002, the Magnet Recognition Program, initiated in 1994, has endorsed 69 institutions that provide the "very best" nursing care. Institutions that apply for magnet status proceed through a rigorous evaluation process based on quality indicators and standards of practice as defined in the ANA's Scope and Standards for Nursing Administrators (**www.nursecredentialing.org/magnet/index.html**).

Outcome Criteria

Stakeholder Satisfaction

Health care organizations have many stakeholders with a vested interest in their own satisfaction as well as in the perceived status of the organization. Not surprisingly, research has demonstrated a correlation between employee satisfaction and patient/client satisfaction.

Patient/Client and Family

Most organizations conduct patient satisfaction surveys in order to determine the perception of the "goodness" of the services they provide to and for patients. Organizational leaders are sometimes surprised that their definition of "quality" and that of the patient/family differ from one another. For example, suppose Hospital A has the best outcome for cardiovascular surgery (96%), but the perception of service is in the mid-range (76%) on the most recent patient satisfaction survey. Suppose, on the other hand, that Hospital B falls 10 points short of Hospital A on surgical outcomes (86%), but far surpasses Hospital A on services (97%).

In the minds of the public, service and quality are indistinguishable. As some have noted, "We expect your clinical practice to be excellent; we want exceptional service, too. We can 'see' the service and to us that means quality."

Organizations also conduct surveys of people in the community who do not use their services. In this way, they are able to determine if the perception of "strangers" is similar to or different from those familiar with the institution. The results of such surveys may be used in creating or revising the organization's marketing plan.

While well-meaning staff members and managers may conduct informal satisfaction surveys at the unit level, a word of caution is in order. The survey results that "count" are those that are derived from the use of valid, reliable survey instruments and processes. The Press Ganey Survey is widely used by health care institutions throughout the United States.

Staff and Physicians

As with patient satisfaction surveys, organizations periodically "take the pulse" of staff members and physicians. For some facilities, a high rate of physician satisfaction translates to an improved bottom line.

Results of staff satisfaction surveys identify areas of focus for managers who are interested in improving the workplace environment. Again, a word of caution is in order. Suppose there are 140 employees on a given unit who care for the unit's patients seven days a week, 24 hours per day. All were given the opportunity to complete a satisfaction survey. A total of 12 surveys were returned, all of them from the night shift. The greatest source of dissatisfaction has to do with the hours of work. Those who responded to the survey indicated a preference for an 11:00 p.m. to 7:00 a.m. rotation, rather than the 12 midnight to 8:00 a.m. rotation that has been in place for several years. The manager most likely has a great deal more work to do before acting on this finding.

Payers

Payers, too, are stakeholders with a keen interest in the status of the organizations with which they contract. Payer satisfaction has to do with value for their investment and satisfaction on the part of their employees with the care and service provided. Certainly payers are interested in the organization's quality outcomes, but benefit coordinators want to know that employees receive timely, high quality care that keeps them well and productive in the job setting or healthy in their retirement.

Report cards

Industry report cards issued by accrediting bodies such as those mentioned above or by private or quasi-governmental "watchdog" agencies are part of doing business in today's quality-conscious environment. Report cards compare facilities or organizations with one another or show how agencies compare with pre-established industry benchmarks.

Institutions that want to truly excel in the area of quality may wish to avail themselves of the tools and techniques offered by such organizations as the Institute for Healthcare Improvement and the national Institute for Standards and Technology, specifically the Baldrige Criteria for Performance Excellence (in Health Care).

Benchmarking

Benchmarking is a technique that identifies "best in class" as a means of comparing one's practice or institution with those who are judged objectively to be the standard-bearer or pacesetter in a given category. For example, the magnet hospital project highlights those institutions that meet or exceed the highest standards for patient care; outcomes of care; and staff retention, involvement, and satisfaction.

Internal benchmarks may identify a particular department with a consistently excellent track record.

A brief word of caution relative to benchmarking: Benchmark achievements are often published and others are challenged or admonished to achieve the same outcomes as the benchmark company or department without benefit of learning about the process the benchmark facility went through to achieve its esteemed status. It is in learning about the process that people or institutions gain the most insight about what creates success for those that others hope to emulate.

Functional Status

Functional areas within the organization include production, marketing, distribution, human resources, marketing, finance, and research and development. The extent to which each functional unit accurately performs the work for which it is accountable, the better positioned the organization is to achieve its goals and surpass its competitors. Functional areas are interdependent; a failure to achieve intended results in one area may cause problems in another area. For example, suppose the organization is known for its excellence in care of patients undergoing invasive cardiovascular surgery. Marketing conducts an aggressive ad campaign at the same time four (out of 11) of the most expert cardiovascular surgical nurses are planning to retire within the next six weeks with no replacements in sight despite the fact that human resources has been "beating the bushes" for months. Unless representatives of the various functional areas are in constant communication with one another and continually evaluate their overlapping strategies with an eye on the whole of the organization, minor or major calamities are inevitable.

1

RESEARCH

Conducting Research

Research is critical to the growth of any profession. Here are a number of reasons why nurses should be able to use and understand research and statistical methods:

- To read the literature and studies with scrutiny and apply findings to their work;
- To conduct applied research relevant to patient needs;
- To move nursing from the artistic and intuitive toward the deliberative and tested so that care at the bedside is based on solid knowledge coupled with the compassion that is inherent in nursing;
- To move nursing closer to the other applied health fields that are research based and in this way develop more collaborative relationships with colleagues in other health care disciplines

Research can be categorized in the following manner:

- **Applied research** — research designed to solve a practical problem or to answer an immediate question.
- **Basic research** — research designed to test and evaluate theories or to contribute to a body of knowledge.
- **Case study research** — research that involves intensive study or investigation of a single individual or group.
- **Descriptive research** — research that describes or reports selected variables and seeks to prove (to others) that facts already accepted really exist; no hypotheses are tested.
- **Developmental research** — research that deals with changes that occur as a result of maturation or development.
- **Experimental research** — research in which participants are randomly assigned to experimental and control groups, an independent variable is manipulated, and scores on a dependent variable are measured, leading to conclusions about the effect of the independent variable upon the dependent variable.
- **Field research** — research conducted in the real world or in a natural setting.
- **Historical research** — research designed to explain or interpret particular phenomena that happened in the past.
- **Laboratory research** — research conducted in a setting specifically designed for research.
- **Longitudinal research** — developmental research that involves measuring the same individuals at various times as they grow older.
- **Qualitative research** — research that does not follow the scientific model and that focuses on the collection and subjective interpretation of data rather than on the testing of a theory.

Data gathering is an important element of any research endeavor. Data are qualitative or quantitative.

- **Qualitative data** — think words! Descriptions in narrative form: concepts, facts, verbatim statements from participants, subjective observations.
- **Quantitative data** — think numbers! Quantification enhances the precision of studies. Data are categorized in the following ways:
  - *Nominal data* — categorical; cannot be arranged in any order with respect to one another. Examples: marital status, religious affiliation, political affiliation.
  - *Ordinal data* — categories are ordered, but differences cannot be determined or they are meaningless. Data can be arranged in some order. Examples: socioeconomic status (lower middle, middle, or upper middle classes), car sizes (compact, midsize, luxury), restaurant/ hotel ratings (one star, two star, five star, etc), or survey questionnaires where the respondent is asked to rank order selected choices.
  - *Interval/ratio data* — interval and ratio level data have categories that are ordered; meaningful differences can be determined. With ratio data there is an absolute zero. With interval data there is no absolute zero. Ratio data are considered a subset of interval data. Examples of interval data: temperature, time (Gregorian calendar measurements), or survey questionnaires using known intervals (as with Likert-type scales). Examples of ratio data: age, weight, height, or distance. Ratio and interval data measure relationships or differences.

Instruments and methods used to gather data must be **valid, reliable, and usable.**

- **Validity** means that the data-gathering instrument measures what it is supposed to measure. It is the most important characteristic of a measuring device. Validity is never 100%; something always falls short. However, it is important to determine if the validity of an instrument is sufficient to be used for the purpose of the particular study under investigation.
- **Reliability** means how well and how consistently an instrument measures something. Most instruments are not perfect and their reliability is expressed as a coefficient number with 1.00 equal to 100%. A correlation coefficient equal to or greater than .80 is considered an acceptable level of reliability. The degree of reliability is determined by the purpose for which the instrument is used.
- An instrument may be reliable (able to measure something consistently) without being valid (appropriate instrument for the measures desired). But an instrument may not be considered valid unless it has both reliability and validity—it must measure consistently and accurately what it is supposed to measure.
- No matter how well the research question is formulated or the hypothesis generated, the outcome of a study depends on the appropriateness of measures used, their validity and reliability, and the extent to which effective, useful data-analysis techniques can make the findings meaningful and useful for their intended purpose.

- Pre-testing of self-developed instruments is a must! Pre-testing on a population sample similar to the one planned for the study is essential. Evaluating the strengths and weaknesses of an instrument and making needed revisions assures proper use of the data-gathering tool. "Pilot study" is another term for pre-testing.

Study Population and Sampling

The term "population" is used to define the group to be studied.

- **Target population** — individuals or things that meet the criteria of interest to the investigator.
- **Sample population** — a miniature version of the target population. This is the group that is usually available to use in a study, and who meet the criteria of the target population.

Sampling concepts include:

- **Random sampling** — all members of the population have an equal chance of being included in the study.
- **Probability sampling** — the investigator can specify for each element of the population the probability that it will be included in the sample. Sample units are selected by chance, and neither investigator nor the population elements have any conscious influence on the constitution of the final sample. Simple random sampling, stratified random sampling, or cluster sampling are considered part of this category.
- **Non-probability sampling** — the investigator has no ability to estimate the probability that each element of the population can or will be a part of the sample, or even that it has a chance of being included. Non-probability samples do not permit generalization beyond the current study group. Confounding factors may influence this type of sampling more than a random sampling, thus making use of findings of less potential value to a broader population.
    - *Convenience sampling* — "accident sampling" — simply taking those people who are available in the right place at the right time.
    - *Purposive sampling* — "judgment sampling" — investigator establishes certain criteria and selects subjects according to these criteria.
    - *Quota sampling* — similar to convenience sampling, but with controls to prevent overloading with subjects having certain characteristics.
- **Sample size** — determined by the number (N) that can logically be included, are available, and that suits the purpose of the study for precision, target population size, desirability for generalization beyond the study group, and importance of the outcomes for decision making. Rule of thumb: use a large enough sample to be representative of the target population; use the largest group possible within the constraints of the study. In general, the larger the sample, the less error there is in measurement and the more significant the findings. An N of less than 30–45 subjects reduces the ability to use strong, powerful statistical analysis of the data.

1

- **Correlation** — means the relationship between two or more factors or characteristics. Correlation is often spoken of as "positive" or "negative" in relation to a numerical coefficient. Critically important concept: correlation of factors with one another in no way proves causation! Though cause and effect relationships are often implied, such assumptions are often erroneous and cannot be substantiated by statistical analysis.

Measures of Central Tendency and Dispersion

The mean, median, and mode are all measures of central tendency, the purpose of which is to isolate one response that is representative of the sample. In some cases, the mean, median, and mode may be identical to one another.

- **Mean** — the average score of the sample; used with interval or ratio data. Method: total the scores of the sample, then divide the total by the number of scores in the sample.
- **Median** — that point in the scale with half the total scores above the point and half the total scores below the point; used with ordinal data or any rating scale.
- **Mode** — the category that occurs with the greatest frequency; the only appropriate measurement for nominal data.

Dispersion, or the degree to which subjects are distanced from the mean, is captured in a measure known as **standard deviation** (SD). This measure requires interval or ratio data. Standard deviation is described as the "average of the averages." It is the most stable measure of variability, that is, the measure of the distance from the mean. SD is a mathematical construct calculated in the following manner:

- Compute the deviation of each raw score from the mean;
- Square and then sum the deviation scores;
- Divide the sum by the number of scores (N) or by N minus one (N – 1);
- Compute the square root of the sum;
- The figure thus arrived at is the SD.

A practical example (for illustrative purposes only; all subtleties of the mathematical model are not included here):

- Suppose there are 100 patients with diabetes who have had an HgbA1C blood test performed within the past month. The mean value of the HgbA1C test results is 7.5, with a range of 6 to 14.5. The care team wants to know the value of the SD. The formula is applied and the SD is calculated as ± 1.5. This means that 68% of the patients have a HgbA1C that is one SD (1.5) from the mean, or 7.5 ± 1.5 (6.0–9.0). Another 28% have a HgbA1C that is two SDs (3.0) from the mean, or 7.5 ± 3.0 (4.5–10.5), and only 4% of patients in the study have HgbA1C readings that are three or more SDs from the mean. If the SD were smaller, e.g., 0.5, the "spread" would be narrower. Conversely, if the SD were larger, e.g., 2.0, the "spread" would be wider.

Hypothesis

The hypothesis is an educated guess. It is the researcher's statement of an expected outcome based on his/her rationale and the design of the study. Hypotheses need be present only in scientific research studies. Generally, there are independent and dependent variables in a hypothesis.

- **Independent variable** — considered to be the cause; occurs first.
- **Dependent variable** — considered to be the effect; depends on and occurs after the independent variable.

  Example: The turnover rate for nurses is greater under authoritarian leadership.

- "Turnover" is the dependent variable — it is affected when the independent variable is added.
- "Authoritarian" is the independent variable — it affects (causes) the turnover rate.

Utilizing Findings

Nursing has been criticized for its failure to vigorously pursue research and to incorporate the findings from research into practice. Until recently, research in nursing was considered an academic endeavor, conducted by those with advanced degrees, and was seen as having little practical application. This mindset took hold despite the fact that Florence Nightingale is recognized as a pioneer in the field of health research and was the first woman to be elected a fellow of the Statistical Society. The value of research in the practice setting is now known and is supported through the establishment of nursing research committees whose members include nurses from all educational backgrounds and from a variety of clinical areas.

Facilitating Research

Many organizations, even those without academic affiliation, now sponsor nursing research committees, provide assistance with grant writing, and educate staff about the value and process of research. Leaders should, to the extent possible, foster research in their institutions and thus contribute to nursing's growing body of research-based knowledge.

Writing Grants

Academic institutions and larger health care systems employ grant writers who are responsible for identifying sources of grants, skillfully crafting the grant proposal, and guiding it through the grant process. Grant-writing workshops are available in most geographical locations or from reputable institutions through the Internet for those who would like to learn more about the process and the availability of grants.

1

Organizations sometimes offer modest, restricted grants that provide the novice grant writer an opportunity to develop a modest research project and apply for funds to carry it out within her/his organizational setting.

Certain private charities, most notably the Pew Charitable Foundation and the Robert Wood Johnson Foundation, offer grants for a wide range of health care endeavors. The U.S. government underwrites millions of dollars in grants each year. Drug companies are exceedingly liberal in providing grant monies, so much so that an obligation to disclose association is now a requirement of any function that may be sponsored by these same companies.

Protection of Human Subjects

The protection of human subjects is of great concern to all of those involved in research. Institutional review boards (IRBs) exist to assure that participants in research studies are protected from unethical practices and unscrupulous researchers.

HIPAA regulations governing research are of interest in a variety of settings. A comprehensive discussion of HIPAA rules that apply to research is beyond the scope of this text. Suffice it to say that HIPAA regulations add a layer of protection to the manner in which data produced by healthcare institutions can be accessed, analyzed and reported. In addition, practitioners engaged in research must become fully aware of, and comply with, HIPAA regulations concerning privacy authorization (**http://privacyruleandresearch.nih.gov/pr_02.asp**).

Ethical Conduct

The National Institutes of Health (NIH) requires all members of its 14 Institutional Review Boards to successfully complete a computer-based training (CBT) program as part of their affiliation with NIH. NIH makes the CBT program available, at no charge, to others. A number of health care organizations involved with human subjects research take advantage of the availability of the CBT program for their own staff members. The program focuses on the clinicians' responsibility to remain above reproach when involved with research having to do with the health and welfare of those they have committed to serve.

CHAPTER 2

Economics

BUDGET

Budget Types: Revenue, Expense, Capital, Operating

The budget categories that managers deal with on an ongoing basis fall primarily into the following categories: revenue, expense, capital, and operating.

The budget is a quantitative statement, usually expressed in monetary terms, of the plans and expectations of a defined entity (company, department, unit) over a specified time period.

Revenue

Revenue is the total amount of income anticipated during a defined period of time. Income sources include reimbursement for patient care, income from goods and products sold, income from membership dues in the case of direct-member health maintenance organizations. Revenue generation is rarely under the direct control of managers. A certain percent of actual or anticipated revenue is allocated to the various cost centers under the manager's direction. The manager is responsible for operating within the revenue allocation by controlling expenses or by creating services that will generate revenue. The extent to which the manager can control fixed expenses is generally limited. Thus, s/he exerts the greatest influence on fiscal stability by controlling variable expenses, including payroll costs.

Expense

The expense budget is comprised of salary and non-salary items. In general, managers are responsible for managing expenditures within assigned **cost** centers (implies outflow of resources/cash). In some settings, managers may also be responsible for a **profit** center (implies inflow of cash).

Costs are describes as fixed and variable. **Fixed** costs are those that remain constant for the organization despite fluctuations in activity levels. Rental fees, contract fees, and insurance premiums are examples of fixed costs. **Variable** costs are costs that fluctuate in response to some internal or external influence such as changes in census, changes in patient acuity, changes in staff mix, or a change in product cost.

Capital

The capital budget includes equipment and renovation expenses needed to meet long-term goals. Organizations define criteria for items included in the capital budget. In general, capital items must have an expected lifespan (performance) of one year or more and exceed a certain dollar value. When budgeting for capital items, costs other than the item itself must be taken into consideration. Such items include: installation costs, delivery charges, service contracts, and so forth.

Managers are expected to know and understand the capital budgeting process for their organization. Amortization is part of the capital process but is often overlooked by managers during the budgeting process. Knowing the "life expectancy" of equipment, programs, or services is critically important so that a replacement strategy can be built into the capital budgeting process. While it is not always possible to predict the rate of obsolescence of a given product or to know what replacement technology is on the horizon, it behooves most managers to gain a greater understanding of the capital process than they currently possess. Those managers who do not have a formal background in finance are well advised to develop working relationships with analysts and controllers in the finance department or to take advantage of participation in a formal budget basics course. In this way, they can gain valuable fiscal management skills.

On a larger scale, capital planning is used to predict and plan for the environmental needs of an organization, that is, the buildings and space the organization requires to conduct its business. The regulatory requirements that surround building plans are such that a relatively long lead time is required. As the delivery of health care and the technology used in its delivery has changed rapidly and significantly in recent years, the traditional planning process has taken on new urgency and faces difficult challenges. In some cases, buildings constructed to house designated clinical services have become outdated even before they are opened because the rate of technology innovation has outstripped the building schedule.

Operating

The operating budget (annual budget) is based on anticipated revenues and expenses for the organization's fiscal year (12 months, not necessarily in concert with the calendar year). Revenue and expense segments are separated; this allows for easy calculation of "bottom line" profit or loss. The operating budget is revisited throughout the year to determine if the organization is on target to meet its projected financial goals. Management practices have a significant impact on the operating budget.

Other — Terminology

The following budgetary terms are part of the leader's financial lexicon:

- **Assets** — the financial resources an organization receives, such as accounts receivable.
- **Break-even point** — the point at which revenue covers cost. The break-even point can be determined by dividing the fixed cost by the contribution margin. For example, if the charge for a procedure is $25 and the actual cost of the procedure is $10, the contribution margin is $15. If the fixed cost for the

procedure for a given period of time (e.g., 12 months) is $30,000, then it would be necessary to perform 2,000 procedures to break even. Most hospitals have high fixed costs.

- **Capital budget** — long-range planning tool for organizations; replacement items budgeted under capital generally have a one- to five-year lifespan.

- **Case mix** — this term refers to the types of patients served by an institution. Case mix is usually defined by variables such as diagnosis, payment source, personal characteristics, and patterns of treatment.

- **Cash flow** — the rate at which dollars are received and disbursed.

- **Centers for Medicare and Medicaid Services (CMS)** — formerly known as the Health Care Financing Administration (HCFA), CMS is the federal agency responsible for implementing Medicare and Medicaid reimbursement regulations. In its reorganized state, CMS has three distinct areas of responsibility: the Center for Medicare Management, the Center for Beneficiary Choices, and the Center for Medicaid and State Operations.

- **Contribution margin** — portion of the charge (to a patient) for a procedure or for supplies that is over and above the actual cost and which the cost center contributes to revenue. For example, if a procedure costs $10 and the patient is charged $25, the contribution margin is $15. The contribution margin is the profit that is contributed by a cost center without the indirect costs.

- **Cost-benefit ratio** — numerical relationship between the value of an activity or procedure in terms of benefits and the value of the activity's cost. The cost-benefit ratio is expressed as a fraction. If the fraction is greater than one (1), benefits outweigh costs, i.e., the activity is economically beneficial.

- **Cost center** — smallest functional unit for which cost control and accountability can be assigned. A nursing unit or floor is usually referred to as a cost center, but there may be other cost centers within a unit (e.g., Orthopedics is a cost center, but often the cast room is considered a separate cost center within Orthopedics).

- **Cost finding** — process of determining full cost of services or procedures by allocating indirect costs and adding them together with direct costs.

- **Diagnostic-related groups (DRGs)** — medical classifications under which a Medicare patient's diagnosis will be made. Each DRG has a set payment reimbursement rate. This rate may, in actuality, be higher or lower than the cost of treating a patient in a particular institution.

- **Direct costs** — costs attributed to a specific source, such as medications and treatments.

- **Endowments** — resources contributed by a donor, but which are held aside to generate additional income for a hospital. For example, a piece of real estate might be donated to a hospital to produce income.

- **Expendable supplies** — supplies that are consumed as used and therefore are not reusable.

- **Fixed budget** — style of budgeting based on a fixed annual level of volume, such as number of patient days or tests performed, to arrive at an annual budget total. Totals are then divided by 12 to arrive at a monthly average. The fixed budget does not make provision for monthly or seasonal variations.

- **Fixed costs** — costs that do not vary according to volume. Examples of fixed costs are mortgage or loan payments.

2

- **Flexible budget** — budgeting system that takes into account variations in volume. Range of activity is estimated based on a projected range of volume from low to high.
- **Forecasting** — process by which future activities are translated into resource needs (persons, supplies, and equipment), which are then translated into dollar amounts.
- **Full cost** — total of all direct and indirect costs.
- **Full-time equivalent (FTE)** — number of hours of work for which a full-time employee is scheduled for a weekly period. For example, 1.0 FTE = five eight-hour days of staffing, which equals 40 hours of staffing per week. One FTE can be divided in different ways. For example, two part-time employees, each working 20 hours per week, would equal I.0 FTE. If a position requires coverage for more than five days or 40 hours a week, the FTE will be greater than 1.0 for that position. If a position requires seven-day coverage for more than five days (or 40 hours) a week, the FTE will be greater than 1.0 for that position. If a position requires seven-day coverage, or 56 hours, then that position requires 1.4 FTE coverage (56 divided by 40 = 1.4). This means that more than one person is needed to fill the FTE position for a seven-day period.
- **Gross income** — total income received before expenses are deducted.
- **Health Care Financing Administration (HCFA)** — See Centers for Medicare and Medicaid Services.
- **Hours per patient day (HPPD)** — hours of nursing care provided per patient per day by various levels of nursing personnel. HPPD are determined by dividing total production hours by number of patients.
- **Indirect costs** — costs that cannot be directly attributed to a specific area. They are usually spread among different departments. Housekeeping services are considered indirect costs.
- **Inflation factor** — percentage rate of inflation. This figure needs to be included in budgeting for the future.
- **Liabilities** — financial obligations of an organization, such as bills to be paid.
- **Major diagnostic category (MDC)** — major categories under which discreet DRGs fall.
- **Master budget** — total budget for the entire organization. The master budget combines the individual cost center budgets.
- **Net income** — income that remains when expenses have been subtracted from total revenues.
- **Net Loss** — loss sustained when expenses exceed total revenues.
- **Operating expenses** — daily costs required to maintain and run a hospital or other health care institution.
- **Outliers** — under the classification of patients by DRGs, this term refers to inpatients who are atypical and cannot be classified by DRG.
- **Patient classification system** — method of classifying patients. Different criteria are used for different systems. In nursing, patients are usually classified according to severity of illness.
- **Planning** — process by which goals and objectives are set. When planning, it is important to anticipate future problems and to make decisions in advance about how to handle them.

- **Position control plan** — plan for staffing requirements that determines how many FTEs are required to deliver the amount of care identified as being necessary.
- **Preferred provider organization (PPO)** — physician, group of physicians, hospital, or other health care facility that has contracted with private insurance companies or individual businesses to provide health care services.
- **Production hours** — total amount of regular time, overtime, and temporary time. This may also be referred to as actual hours.
- **Profit margin** — percentage difference between expenses and revenue.
- **Program budget** — style of budgeting that involves planning for five or 10 years ahead. Attention is paid to external events that might impact an organization. As long-range plans are determined, specific objectives are identified that will lead to the achievement of the plans. The costs required to meet these objectives are then determined. Alternative objectives and their costs may also be identified in order to provide greater flexibility. Programs are prioritized in order of importance.
- **Restricted resources** — financial contributions that have restrictions placed on their use by the donor. For example, resources donated for specific programs, units, or services are considered restricted.
- **Revenue** — items or amounts of income.
- **Semi-fixed costs** — costs that run at a certain level for a given period of time and then increase. For example, one chef can prepare a certain number of meals at a certain fixed cost. After a certain point, another chef needs to be hired to handle the additional volume.
- **Staffing distribution** — determination of number of personnel allocated per shift. For example: 45% day shift, 35% evening shift, 20% night shift.
- **Staffing mix** — ratio of various types of personnel to one another. For example, a shift on one unit might have 40% RNs, 40% LPNs/LVNs, 20% other.
- **Tax Equity and Fiscal Responsibility Act of 1982 (TEFRA)** — federal act which restricted reimbursement to a predetermined rate for Medicare patients. This regulation was superseded in 1984 by the diagnostic-related group (DRG) method of payment.
- **Turnover rate** — rate at which employees leave their jobs for reasons other than death or retirement. The rate is calculated by dividing the number of employees leaving by the average number of workers employed in the unit during the year and then multiplying by 100.
- **Unrestricted resources** — financial contributions that have no restrictions placed on their use by the donor.
- **Variable costs** — costs that vary with the volume, e.g., payroll costs.
- **Variance** — difference between planned costs and actual costs.
- **Workload index** — weighted statistic that reflects acuity level of patients, census, and production hours. The workload index can serve as a baseline for productivity improvement. One way to determine a workload index is as follows:

$$\frac{\text{Acuity Index X Workload Units}}{\text{Production Hours}}$$

2

- **Zero-based budgeting** — type of budgeting system that starts at zero each year. This means that every dollar to be spent needs to be justified. Established costs are not automatically continued from one year to the next. This style of budgeting ensures that activities are not continued simply because they were carried out in the past. In zero-based budgeting, objectives are important and are listed according to priority. Zero-based budgeting also indicates what will happen if an objective is eliminated, as well as which objectives could be accomplished for less money.

Uses

Budgets, budget reports, and forecasts are used to demonstrate the fiscal responsibility and financial health of an organization. Generated income is placed in the "trust' of the organization with the assumption that the resources will be used wisely and well for their intended purpose.

Development

Budget information is supplied to managers in advance of the annual budget-planning cycle. The information provides a retrospective history of the financial activities and status of the department, unit, or organization. It also shows the anticipated revenue for the coming year, the revenue sources, and any uncertainties related to revenue streams. Optimistic, moderate, and pessimistic scenarios may also be presented as part of the budget development process.

Managers work within a timeline to create preliminary, revised, and final budgets consistent with the practices of the organization. Review and approval procedures are built into the development process all along the line. Therefore, once the final budget is released, there should be no "big" surprises.

Monitoring

Managers are expected to routinely monitor budget reports. In most cases, reports are generated and reviewed on a monthly basis. Managers are asked to justify deviations from the budget predictions and to make adjustments accordingly. In some cases, monthly allocations are divided equally among the months of the year. In other cases, monthly allocations are adjusted based on historical trends. In any case, the manager must become familiar with trends and the trending methodology in use in her/his organization. Failure to consider trends when making interval adjustments to budgets sometimes results in over or under correction of variance and leads to more difficulties downstream.

Justifying

Budget items must be justified, that is, the reason for the expenditure must be clearly known and understood, and it must be consistent with the overall objectives and fiscal plan of the organization. A justification process is in place in most institutions. Depending on the scope of the anticipated expenditure, its sponsor(s) may be requested to submit a business case to justify the item. The organization then prior-itizes requests according to established criteria. In certain circumstances, budget items that initially put the organization or the department into a negative variance are seen as justifiable because the long-term return on investment will yield finan-cial benefit for the organization.

Variance Analysis

Because budgets are fluid, line items are rarely precisely on target. Thus, variance analysis is an essential part of the budget process. If the variance exceeds a predeter-mined target, then further investigation is warranted. (This is so whether the variance is positive or negative.) Variances may be characterized as volume, efficiency, rate, or non-salary expenditures. Volume variances in the hospital setting may occur in response to a fluctuation in patient days. Efficiency variances in the hospital setting may be expressed in changes from the anticipated hours per patient per day. Rate vari-ances reflect the difference between the budgeted hourly rate and the paid hourly rate. Non-salary expenditure variances may be caused by changes in patient mix, patient volume, supply quantities, supply costs, price paid, or new technology or regulations.

Reports

Managers generally receive monthly, quarterly, annual, and predictive budget reports that help them better manage their units or services. In addition, managers should receive reports detailing the overall financial status of the organization. Reports must be reviewed for accuracy and analyzed for hidden content; that is, to learn the "story" behind the numbers. For example, is a high sick rate on a given unit related to outbreak of the flu, interpersonal conflict on the unit, chronic "short staffing," management practices, or "none of the above"?

To the extent possible, managers should receive financial reports "on-line." Such reports may use a simple spreadsheet approach or may be embedded in a more sophis-ticated software program. In either case, managers should know how to interpret and manipulate both paper and electronic budget reports as part of their practice.

Decision Support Systems

Decision support systems allow managers to make financial decisions and adjust-ments through computer modeling that uses real time data. Most institutions now use computer-generated financial forecasting. This methodology allows organiza-tions to develop alternative scenarios based on the interplay among numerous vari-ables. While computer programs are capable of generating an infinite number of sce-narios, it is the wisdom and knowledge of the people in the organization that define the probable scenarios that the organization is likely to face in the near or far term. Astute managers and administrators inform themselves about scenario develop-ment, the availability and capability of computerized forecasting systems, and the process used by the organization in forecast planning.

Unlike strategic planning, scenario development is characterized by a focus on possible futures. The creation of scenarios allows organizations or departments to

2

compensate for errors common in the planning process—under-prediction and over-prediction. The scenarios create focus on an organization's key concerns in areas of uncertainty. For example, suppose that the organization's strategic plan predicts 3–4% growth over each of the next 10 years and bases its resource acquisition on this assumption. The company faces grave consequences in its financial position if growth falls below 2.6% per year on average. Scenario development will help this company examine the possible consequences of excessive growth or excessive loss, each of which is a possibility, neither of which is accounted for in the strategic plan.

REIMBURSEMENT

Revenue streams for health care organizations originate from a variety of sources.

DRGs and PPSs (Diagnosis-Related Groups and Prospective Payment Systems)

Diagnosis-related groups (DRGs) categorize the care needs of hospitalized patients based on primary and secondary diagnosis, age, and treatments provided. There are over 400 DRGs. DRGs came into use in 1983 as a way to deter cost shifting within the Medicare system. The DRG reimbursement rate is fixed and is calculated based on the law of averages. The resources used to care for some patients who fall into a particular category will exceed the reimbursement rate; for others, the cost of care will be less than the reimbursement rate.

The Medicare Prospective Payment System (PPS) is the mechanism for transferring funds to hospitals, based on the facility's DRG profile. Prospective payment schemes provide a predetermined amount of money to the organization based on the anticipated utilization by a defined group of patients.

While DRGs and PPS were initially a system used by the federal government to constrain Medicare costs, it was merely a matter of time before the process was more widely adopted, first by Medicaid and then by private sector insurers. PPS effectively signaled the end of the "usual and customary" reimbursement system based on charges for care/service, rather than on the cost of those services.

Capitation

Capitation is an inherent part of managed care systems. Health maintenance organizations (HMOs), preferred provider organizations (PPOs), and medical service organizations (MSOs) are financed through capitation. In the capitated model, the organization is paid a fixed, negotiated rate per member (life covered) per month

(PM/PM). The organization receives payment whether or not the member uses the services of the organization in a given time period. Organizations financed under capitation are expected to manage their business in such a way that they provide all needed and agreed upon care to the patients covered under the plan.

The business model calls for risk to be spread within the group for the array of services that are agreed upon ahead of time. In general, the care provided is "conservative," that is, the services provided are intended to prevent illness, to maintain health, and to care for episodic acute care needs based on known/proven therapies. The regulations that govern managed care are such that organizations open themselves to considerable risk if they provide care beyond what the plan promises to provide. For example, a request for payment for an experimental treatment that the plan has not yet adopted but that might be of benefit for one member of the plan will be refused. This same treatment may eventually move from experimental to mainstream and be incorporated into the plan's offerings. However, if the plan were to provide the care for the one member who requested it, as noted above, then this same care (procedure, therapy) would need to be offered to others in the plan with a similar condition. The risk model used by the managed care group is then overridden, placing the organization in financial and regulatory jeopardy. This is sometimes a difficult concept for the general public to understand and thus news headlines tend to place the organization in an unfavorable light. It is also true that some unscrupulous organizations have failed to provide the care and services promised under their capitated contracts.

HMOs

The term "health maintenance organization" (HMO) became part of the health care lexicon in 1973 with the passage of the HMO Act. The HMO Act established federal standards for HMOs and required companies of a certain size to offer at least one HMO to their employees. The principles underlying HMOs are cost-effectiveness based on productivity, population management with a focus on preventive care, a predetermined and agreed upon array of services including both ambulatory and inpatient care, prepayment in the form of "dues" or "membership," and assumption of risk by the provider to meet the requirements of the promised care and service.

Prepaid group practice is considered the precursor to HMOs. Prepaid group practices were recommended as long ago as 1932 as the most effective delivery system. Insurers, employers, or others contract with the physician group to provide a predetermined range of benefits to a specific population for a fixed and agreed upon price. Providers in this arrangement put themselves at risk in that they were required to provide the full range of agreed upon services, regardless of whether the cost of benefits exceeded the established rate of payment. Ross-Loos, established in Los Angeles in the 1920s, and Kaiser Permanente, established on the West Coast in the 1930s, are the models for prepaid group practice. In their early days they were considered "outcasts" by the traditional medical establishment. This is no longer the case.

A number of HMO models exist, though recent shakeouts in the health care industry have seen some insurers exiting the HMO market and some excellent programs becoming insolvent due to financial crises.

2

- **Independent (or individual) practice association (IPA)** — open-panel system in which individual physicians or the practice association contract to provide care to enrolled members. Physicians retain their right to treat fee-for-service patients. (Note: many IPAs have ceased existence because they were unable to remain financially viable.)
- **Staff model** — majority of physicians are on the staff of, and derive their salary from, the HMO; physicians on staff are sole or major source of care for enrollees.
- **Group model** — single large multi-specialty group is sole or major source of care for enrollees; contract is exclusively with one HMO. (Note: because of the similarity in the staff and group models, the label "staff/group model" is often used.)
- **Network model** — two or more group practices contract to care for the majority of patients enrolled in an HMO plan. The physicians are usually able to care for fee-for-service patients as well as HMO patients.

Constraints apply to those who receive care through HMO systems. Unless they are willing to pay out-of-pocket, members receive care from providers who contract with or who are employed by the HMO. The same is true for choice of hospitals. These limits are generally offset by the array of services provided, the relative lower cost of managed care plans, and the reasonable co-payments that some patients pay at the point of care.

Market share for HMOs tends to be geographical in nature with significant penetration in metropolitan areas on the East and West Coasts and in a few markets in the interior, for example, the Twin Cities corridor (Minneapolis/St. Paul). The extent to which managed care will be adopted in other markets is unknown. Through the 1990s, the assumption was that the HMO approach to care would prevail over time. That certainty is no longer apparent in the face of the collapse of respected programs and a growing pessimism within the medical community, most having to do with reimbursement conflicts under various managed care contracts.

SHMOs

The social health maintenance organization (SHMO) is a demonstration model conducted under the sponsorship of Medicare to determine the value and feasibility of combining social, health, and medical services under one umbrella with a single payment. Services provided, in addition to those covered under traditional Medicare or Medicaid, include adult day care, dental, vision, hearing, meals, transportation, hospice care, respite care, homemaker services, and chronic care in a nursing facility without prior hospitalization.

A demonstration project, the Program for All-Inclusive Care for the Elderly (PACE), conducted under the auspices of HCFA (Health Care Financing Administration, now CMS, Centers for Medicare and Medicaid Services) replicated the On Lok model in place in San Francisco's Chinatown in several locations throughout the country. The intent was to determine the feasibility of increasing Medicare long-term care (LTC) benefits. Early findings showed that SHMOs were able to reduce hospitalization rates compared with the rates of the non-SHMO Medicare population, but that total costs were not necessarily reduced. All sites experienced substantial losses during the first three years of operation. By year five, two projects broke even or experienced modest gains; the other two sustained losses.

A recent report assesses two generations of social HMOs (S/HMO I and S/HMO II). S/HMO I plans are in Brooklyn, NY; Portland, OR; and Long Beach, CA. The S/HMO II is in Las Vegas/Reno, NV. Only one of the three S/HMO I plans examined has implemented innovative geriatric approaches. However, costs for the S/HMO I plans are 15–27% higher than they would have been had the plans been paid under the same formula as traditional Medicare HMOs. The higher payments appear unwarranted for two of the three plans, because their enrollees are no frailer than comparably aged enrollees in local Medicare HMOs. Furthermore, plans report spending less than the full supplementary payment on the extra services the supplement was intended to cover. The S/HMO II plan, a newer model, also has implemented innovative geriatric programs and is not overpaid relative to the health of its enrollees.

Despite the enhanced services, member satisfaction with the four S/HMOs is about the same as for regular Medicare HMOs in the same cities. The most innovative of the S/HMOs—the S/HMO II plan—does not appear to have a greater effect than regular HMOs on beneficiaries' health and functioning. Given these findings, the authors of the report recommend that the S/HMO plans be phased into the regular Medicare+Choice program by 2007, and that the special payment method be phased out.

Negotiating Capitated Discount Rates

During the budgeting process, health care organizations assess various income streams, including a review of capitated contracts. In the presence of a guaranteed income for an agreed upon set of services for a given population group, the organization may agree to the payer's request for a discounted rate. Before such an agreement is reached, the organization must determine how much risk it is willing to accept in order to set the discount rate. For example, suppose the capitated rate for Group A is set at X dollars per member, per month. Group A is considered a moderate risk group, is mixed in age, and has a history of reasonable use of services. Group B, on the other hand, is composed of young, healthy members with very low utilization and no chronicity. The benefits coordinator for Group B wants to negotiate a lower rate, preferably with no increase in co-pays for Group B members. The organization must determine if it can sustain the risk and agree to a steeper discounted rate for Group B. If it does agree in principle, then the co-payment issue must still be addressed.

In the current market, "low rate, high deductible" products are becoming popular with payers and members alike. Members who opt for these products generally see themselves as being in excellent health and in need of very little in the way of health care services. They reason, and employers/payers may concur, that the lowest-cost plan is their best choice. The decision seems reasonable until such a time as the "law of averages" takes hold and the "healthy" individual suffers a catastrophic accident or experiences an unexpected illness and is faced with a devastatingly high "co-pay."

2

PPO

Preferred provider organizations (PPOs) came into being in response to discontent with other models of managed care. The PPO is an integrated system in which the PPO serves as a broker between the purchaser of care and the provider. In a PPO, clients have the option to use or not use the preferred providers available in the plan. In-plan providers are generally considered more "attractive" to clients because of lower costs and greater benefits. Providers are paid a discounted fee-for-service and do not participate in financial risk sharing.

Though the PPO affords the client greater choice than a staff model HMO, its ability to control costs is limited by the level of discount that can be negotiated with providers.

Traditional Third-Party Payers

Third-party payers do not provide any direct care; rather, they pay providers/provider groups to care for defined groups or individuals. The U.S. government is the largest third-party payer. It is the exclusive payer for traditional Medicare and funds Medicaid at varying rates depending on contributions negotiated state by state. A significant number of Medicare and Medicaid contracts are now negotiated as managed care contracts.

Traditional indemnity insurance offers the greatest freedom and flexibility. Those covered by such a plan can choose to receive care from any primary care or specialist physician or go to the hospital of their choosing at any time. They can also change physicians or hospitals at will. The insurance company pays for the majority of care received in an acute care facility and pays varying amounts for outpatient services depending on the buyer's choice of plan. For example, healthy young people are likely to choose a high deductible plan in which they will pay out-of-pocket for the majority of outpatient care received in a given year. The out-of-pocket costs are offset by the lower insurance premiums. On the other hand, someone who has chronic, ongoing health problems will choose a lower deductible and pay a higher premium. In some cases, the premiums for people with pre-existing health conditions are prohibitively high, or they may not qualify for indemnity insurance at all, even if they are able to pay the premiums. A number of insurance companies, for example, Blue Cross/Blue Shield, offer HMO, PPO, and indemnity plans.

Medicare
(See additional remarks about Medicare under "Legal and Regulatory Issues.")

The Medicare program was created in 1965 to pay for health services for people age 65 and older. Medicare originated through Title XVIII of the Social Security Act. Though it was initially aimed at the retirement age population (at the time of its passage age 65 was the mandatory retirement age as well as the age for Social Security eligibility), Medicare was expanded in 1972 to include people of any age with end-stage renal disease (i.e., those receiving dialysis). In 1973 it was expanded to include people of any age who meet Medicare's definition of disability. Ninety percent of Medicare beneficiaries are age 65 and above.

Medicaid

(See additional remarks about Medicaid under "Legal and Regulatory Issues.")

As with Medicare, the Medicaid program was established in 1965 and implemented in 1966. Medicaid is defined as a welfare program that pays for certain mandated health services provided to low-income children and their caretakers. Generally, the caretakers receive, or are eligible to receive, public assistance funds. Until 1996 these funds were administered through Aid to Families with Dependent Children (AFDC). The Personal Responsibility and Work Opportunity Reconciliation Act of 1996 (PL 104–93) replaced AFDC with the Temporary Assistance for Needy Families (TANF) program. Over time amendments to the Medicaid act have been made to include people with developmental disabilities and other low-income groups, including the elderly, children, and pregnant women.

Medicaid is funded jointly by the federal and state governments. The state's per capita income determines the amount of federal matching funds.

Insurance

Indemnity insurance is the traditional method of obtaining health insurance for an array of services that are generally needed only under extraordinary circumstances. Indemnity insurance generally covers a predetermined percentage of acute care services, regardless of the absolute charge for those services. For example, two clients pay the same fixed monthly amount for their insurance based on similarity in their risk factors. One needs a hysterectomy and goes to Hospital A for the procedure. Hospital A charges $2,000 for the care provided. The client's insurance carrier pays 80% of the bill, or $1,600. The client is then responsible for the additional $400. The other client has the same procedure at Hospital B, but the charges are $3,000. Again, the client's insurance carrier pays 80% of the bill, or $2,400, but in this case the client's out-of-pocket expense is $600.

There are numerous varieties of indemnity insurance. In a "tight" economy that finds employers less willing or able to pay high insurance premiums for employees, or in which more people must assume responsibility for their own insurance coverage, "low premium, high deductible" plans are offered as a product line. The impact of such products on the health care industry is not yet known.

COST CONTAINMENT

The cost of health care continues to outstrip the rate of inflation by several percentage points each year. The forces that drive costs higher are well known; they include the aging of the population and the burden of chronic disease, the cost of technology, the cost of pharmaceuticals, the rising expectations of the public about the capabilities of the health care system, and lifestyle choices. By the same token, the health care industry has lagged in its adoption of efficiencies apparent in other large-scale enterprises. Some industry watchers suggest that health care costs could be significantly reduced if the industry applied proven efficiency measures to its practices. A variety of interventions have been attempted or are in place to staunch the ever-increasing dollar amount spent on health care. The degree to which these measures are succeeding is unknown; "voluntary" measures attempted in the past, such as the Professional Review Organizations (PROs), were considered a failure. It is possible that some measures now in place are working even as the cost of care continues to rise. Some analysts suggest that, in the absence of these measures, costs would rise even more rapidly!

Here, briefly outlined, are a number of approaches to cost containment.

Managed Care

"Managed care" is an amorphous term, not unlike "quality care"! Still, most would agree that a central concept of managed care is the integration, at some level, of the financing and delivery of care. Patient utilization and provider practices are overseen by an entity than has a fiduciary interest in the interactions between the two.

Advocates of managed care expect that it will:

- Optimize the use of resources, avoiding overuse or under use;
- Increase accountability at all levels;
- Accurately predict expenditures;
- Contain or reduce expenditures;
- Shift focus from acute care and crisis intervention to disease prevention and health maintenance;
- Reduce variation in practice;
- Ensure better outcomes of care.

Full realization of the ideals listed above remains elusive even in the best of managed care systems; progress is slow. To its detractors, the term "managed care" is regarded with disdain, the concept is considered a failure, and the impact is seen as a "take away."

Models of managed care have been described above (i.e., HMOs, SHMOs, and so forth).

Cost-Benefit Analysis

Cost-benefit analysis is the process of examining scenarios to determine the relative value of an intervention when measured against predetermined criteria. For example, is it more or less cost effective to provide home care or to pay for care in a skilled nursing facility? Is it more or less cost effective to care for indigent patients in the emergency department than to establish a community clinic? While the answers to these dilemmas may seem intuitive, they are not; nor is the process of analysis, because human lives are at stake and the emotions of the decision makers, not to mention the target populations, come into play.

While traditional cost-benefit analysis techniques have been used in health care for many years, more sophisticated systems are now being introduced. One such approach is known as the Archimedes simulation model. According to researchers involved with Archimedes, this system "takes advantage of the latest advantages in computing, software design and mathematical modeling" to replicate the reality of the practice world. Archimedes includes all aspects of care—faculties, personnel, care processes, protocols, logistics and costs, multiple disease conditions, and needed interventions over time. Biomathematical modeling allows analysts to address complex problems rapidly and inexpensively, in contrast to other methods such as clinical trials, observational studies, or the judgment of experts. The extent to which biomathematical modeling achieves its promise is yet to be determined.

Productivity

Productivity is an industrial term that describes the relationship between "outputs" (products delivered) and "inputs" (the resources utilized to produce the outputs). Whether or not the traditional concept of productivity can be applied to complex systems such as health care remains a subject for debate.

The Agency for Healthcare Research and Quality (AHRQ), formerly known as the Agency for Healthcare Policy and Research (AHCPR), commissioned Patient Outcome Research Teams (PORTS) to answer critical questions about the effectiveness and cost effectiveness of available treatments for common clinical conditions. The first PORTs began their work in 1989.

> The PORTs were designed to take advantage of readily available data and to focus on common clinical conditions that are costly to the Medicare and Medicaid programs and for which there is regional variability in outcomes and use of resources. The PORTs are made up of a multidisciplinary team of researchers ranging from health economists and clinicians to quality-of-life experts and epidemiologists. PORT investigators were instructed to answer the following questions: What works and at what cost? For which patients or subgroups of patients? When? Why is there variation in the use of treatments? What can be done to reduce inappropriate variation? From whose perspective—i.e, the patient is the ultimate judge of effectiveness? Is there a potential for development and use of patient-reported outcome measures?.

Specific to the field of nursing, two models of productivity are briefly described here. The first is the **industrial model** that measures the ratio of work output to work input (efficiency). Nursing hours per patient per day or costs per unit of service are examples of the industrial model based on principles of the school of scientific management that came into its own in the 1920s. The second is the **systems framework,** which embraces both efficiency and effectiveness. In this model, effectiveness includes quality and appropriateness; efficiency includes nursing output with minimal waste. The second model takes into consideration the special characteristics of nursing, such as caring.

- Nursing hours per patient per day (HPPD) = divide total paid hours for nursing personnel for a specific time period by the total number of patient days in the same time period.
- Salary costs per patient per day = divide total payroll expenses for nursing personnel for a specific time by the total number of patient days in the same timeframe (more sensitive measure than HPPD in that it accounts for staff mix).

2

- Utilization rate = required hours of care divided by nursing hours paid. Greater sensitivity in that hours of care required are based on a patient classification system. Results show differences, if any, between the required and actual staffing ratios.

Patient/Client Classification

Classification systems assign patients to defined categories by care intensity, care level, assumed or average utilization of resources, or other variables.

Health care systems may devise their own patient classification systems; however, the tools they use must be valid and reliable. Alternatively, a number of commercial classification systems are readily available for purchase. The purchase of an acuity system package is accompanied by support service from the product's creator or vendor. All commonly available acuity systems are automated.

DRGs are actually a classification system related to reimbursement based on intensity of need. The acronym "DRG" is a now familiar term that stands for "diagnostic-related group." DRGs originated in 1983 as part of the Medicare Prospective Payment System (PPS), which pays care institutions a set amount ahead of time for care rendered for patients with specific conditions. DRG/PPS was initially applied to care provided for Medicare patients in acute care hospitals and was based on the projected case mix for the institution, adjusted for age. Other payers, including Medicaid, and then the private sector, adopted Medicare's approach. PPS has expanded over time and is now applied in other health care settings such as skilled nursing facilities.

PPS was instituted to deter cost shifting. The practice of cost shifting allowed hospitals to recover some uncompensated billings by transferring these costs to Medicare and other payers. With cost shifting no longer an option, hospitals needed to cut costs in order to continue to operate. The intervening years have seen a significant number of hospital closures and consolidation throughout the industry.

An entire sub-industry has now come into play in response to DRGs. Coders, case management enterprises, nurses that specialize in discharge planning and patient placement, publishing companies that produce DRG manuals, and designated government departments now exist to assure compliance with PPS regulations!

Savings related to the advent of DRGs are generally attributed to two factors: decreased lengths of stay in acute care facilities and avoidance of admissions when care can be provided safely in another setting.

Establishing a link between DRG classifications and nursing acuity classification is a challenging but worthwhile endeavor.

Staff Mix

The pattern of assigning defined categories of staff to care for a specific group of patients is known as "staff mix." Depending on the philosophy of the institution, the staff mix may be more or less heavily weighted toward the use of registered nurses. Registered nurses, licensed practical/vocational nurses, and unlicensed assistive personnel (e.g., nurse aides), make up the bulk of a hospital's staff mix for direct care. Other disciplines may assist in the provision of direct or indirect care.

Staffing ratios relative to the use of RNs may be prescribed by legislation, particularly for specialty areas such as intensive care units. RN ratio legislation for other care settings now exists in some states, a trend that is likely to prevail in the coming years. For example, in January 2002, California Governor Gray Davis signed into law a bill mandating minimum nurse-to-patient staffing ratios. Despite legislative intent and institutional commitment, the extent to which staff ratios can be met depends on the availability of registered nurses. And the current nursing shortage is predicted to worsen, at least in the near term.

Critics of staffing ratios maintain that this approach alone is an insufficient guarantee of safe care. Rather, the patient's overall condition, intensity of needs, and requisite competence of the staff must be taken into consideration when determining the optimum staff mix for a particular service.

Reduction in Staff and Services

Costs can be contained through reduction in force (RIF) strategies and the cutback or elimination of services not seen as critical to the organization's goals, including that of maintaining fiscal viability. Outsourcing is another approach to cost reduction. Competitive bids for certain services can be obtained and vendors selected for such services as housekeeping, food, linen, and the like. Payroll, transcription, and other business services can be contracted. Temporary agencies can be used to supplement core staffing, particularly to meet seasonal needs. The relatively high per hour cost of temporary employees may be offset by avoidance of benefit costs. Cost savings achieved by RIFs may not be sustained and hidden costs may outstrip anticipated savings.

Ethical, legal, and contractual issues come into play when RIFs occur. Can the organization's ethical commitment to safe patient care be maintained in the face of downsizing? Does the organization place itself in harm's way by inviting sanctions from regulatory agencies if preventable violations occur? If members of organized labor staff the organization, do contracts include "no layoff" clauses?

Material Management

Economists, efficiency experts, administrators, and frontline staff generally agree that resources can be better managed through the development and application of better business, information, and care systems. In the abstract, there are no arguments about the need to decrease waste in the delivery of health care.

Controlling the cost of supplies and equipment is a never-ending challenge for managers and staff. The process of competitive bidding allows organizations to obtain significant discounts on quality products from various vendors or distributors. While this practice is beneficial to the organization overall, it also tends to isolate staff from the actual cost of materials and supplies in that the cost to the organization is generally closely held information.

2

Inventory control systems help match supply and demand, may decrease utilization, and may decrease loss due to theft. "Pricing" frequently used items may help staff "comparison shop" for the most cost-effective products and supplies even within their own department or institution. Compared with other industries, health care inventory-control systems are still on the upward curve of the improvement process.

In the past, supply costs were "passed through" and reimbursed through the third-party system. Patients as well as staff remained immune to the cost of supplies, which, when itemized, also include the cost of processing.

As with salary and non-payroll personnel costs, managers receive monthly reports detailing materials costs for their units or departments.

MARKETING

Purpose/Market Share/Penetration/Mix

The purpose of marketing is to identify customer needs and meet them in a way that returns value to the organization. The business approach to marketing was once anathema to health care. Whether through formal prohibitions or tradition, health care entities did not market their products and services through usual marketing channels such as advertising and direct-to-consumer approaches. A few short decades ago, physicians or physician groups would have been labeled charlatans for advertising their services. Things have certainly changed!

Through market analysis, health care establishments can determine the existence of potential customers, their needs, the products and services that appeal to target groups, the status of and techniques used by competitors (benchmarking), and what price the market will bear (though there are constraints in this last element for most players in the health care market).

Market penetration refers to how well the organization has exposed its services to potential users and/or buyers. Are the potential buyers aware of the organization, of the products and services it has to offer, of the price of the products and services— and are the products and services appealing to the potential customers? Market share is that portion of the market that is supplied by the organization, for example, how many "lives" a particular provider covers.

Market mix refers to the variety of market segments an organization elects to target (e.g., small businesses, large groups, retirees, women, and children). The term "market mix" can also be applied to the variety and scope of the products or services the organization has to offer to its potential market.

Advertising and the Media

"Brand recognition" happens through advertising. "Brand loyalty" is sustained through advertising. Traditional advertising modalities such as newspapers, televi-

2

sion (including "infomercials"), and radio are expensive. Thus, health care organizations exercise discretion when making decisions to purchase advertising time and space. Most organizations take advantage of "free" publicity; for example, public interest stories that shed a positive light on the organization. Organizations also plan for and evaluate the effectiveness of their advertising campaigns through techniques such as focus groups, surveys, and interviews.

The majority of hospitals and health care systems now have a presence on the Internet. They, along with other health care entities that use the Internet to share information, subscribe to the eHealth code of ethics. Here is eHealth's vision statement: "The goal of the eHealth Code of Ethics is to ensure that people worldwide can confidently and with full understanding of known risks realize the potential of the Internet in managing their own health and the health of those in their care" (www.ihealthcoalition.org/ethics/ehcode.html).

Values expressed in the code include: candor and honesty; quality of information, products, and services; respect for individuals' right to give informed consent; and respect for privacy and protection of confidential information.

Surveys

There is an abundance of market research available to organizations. Most organizations rely on standard market information in addition to their own surveys usually aimed at brand recognition or brand identification. Well-structured, professionally conducted focus groups often provide organizations with useful information that allow them to better target subsequent survey activities.

Image Building

For the organization-at-large: Most organizations have an image they wish to project. The image must be believable, sustainable, honest, and appealing. It should foster loyalty among those who are already part of the organization, or who obtain services from the organization. And it should increase the organization's share of target markets. Once the decision is made to foster a particular image, executive-level efforts should be directed toward assuring that "everyone is on board" with regard to the organization's public persona.

For nursing in particular: Nurses enjoy a highly favorable image among the public at large. However, the public's image of the nurse is still, in many cases, that of a subservient woman who does the bidding of others. The current nursing shortage actually allows nurses to demonstrate the variety, complexity, and significance of their many roles. Interestingly enough, it is more than a bit difficult to describe the deep value of nursing to a general audience, but the challenge is there and the time to meet it, as a profession, is now.

Corporations and foundations: Most notably Johnson & Johnson, through its corporate advertising program and through its philanthropic arm, the Robert Wood

2

Johnson Foundation, is promoting the image and value of nursing to a variety of audiences with the intent of helping to alleviate the serious nursing shortage that will not dissipate any time soon. As of this writing, there are over 120,000 open positions for nurses in the United States.

Public Relations

Organizations employ public relations professionals who interface with the press, with various community constituencies, with law enforcement, with regulatory bodies, with employees, and with patients and families. Their role is to assure consistency in the messages sent to the "outside" world from the organization, to prevent jeopardy to the organization, and to serve as the "voice" of the organization—hopefully in a manner that is seen as enthusiastic, positive, and respectful.

Public relations personnel are sometimes called upon to do "damage control" and must be prepared to absorb or deflect negative comments while maintaining personal dignity and respect for others, even the detractors.

CHAPTER 3

Human Resources

STAFFING

Recruitment

Nurse recruitment occurs in a variety of ways: newspaper advertising, trade journal advertising, strategically placed human-interest stories, the Internet, and television. Perhaps the most effective recruitment strategy is word-of-mouth or person-to-person. Nurses who are satisfied in their current positions are often key to attracting their colleagues to a particular institution. Nurse recruiters, whether or not they themselves are nurses, add a human element to the recruitment process. Many organizations offer bonuses to staff that recruit others to fill particular positions. "Sign on" bonuses are also part of the recruitment strategy.

Retention and Turnover

While recruitment is key to filling positions, purposeful retention strategies are essential to retaining staff once they have joined an organization. Promise keeping is a key ingredient in one's retention strategy. Promises that cannot be kept—for example, every weekend off, no mandatory overtime—should not be made. Honesty breeds respect. Thus, even if employment conditions are less than perfect, a new employee is likely to appreciate the sincerity of the manager who tells the truth about working conditions.

Use of Agency Personnel

Temporary agencies are often used to fill staffing gaps. Organizations may maintain their own "internal registry," contract exclusively with one external agency, use short or long-term "traveler" nurses, or rely on community-based "temp" services to meet their needs.

In union environments, close attention must be paid to the use of temporary agency personnel to assure that conditions of the labor contract are not violated when "temps" are hired.

While agencies are responsible for assuring the quality and competence of temporary staff, the organization in which the temporary staff member practices must also have policies and procedures in place that govern the practice of the "visiting" staff. Of particular importance is the verification of licensure.

Scheduling

Scheduling must be done in such a way that the right persons are available at the right time to care for a defined patient population. Scheduling takes into account "peaks and valleys" that may occur throughout the week or by season. For example, a respiratory care unit is more likely to be filled to capacity in winter months as opposed to summer. Scheduling must also take into account the need to place only qualified staff in a given practice area in order to avoid harm to the patients and/or to the nurse.

Job Analysis

Job analysis is undertaken to systematically define the knowledge and skill needed to perform a particular job and the tasks associated with the job. Job analysis goes beyond the job description and makes the expectations of the position more explicit.

Job Descriptions

Job descriptions include job title, major duties, relationships, educational and/or certification requirements, experience requirements, physical requirements, and work hazards of the job, if any. The job description is written in non-sexist language. Well-written job descriptions help assure that candidates who apply for a particular position are well aware of the scope and limitations of the job. Job descriptions also help recruiters or hiring authorities in the preliminary screening process of potential job candidates.

Role Clarification

Role clarification is a method for determining the expectations two or more people hold of one another in their respective positions. Role clarification may occur proactively when jobs and job responsibilities are changing or shifting in some way. Or it may occur reactively in the presence of conflict or disagreement about scope and responsibility. Role clarification, or role redefinition, is seen as particularly valuable for those moving from staff to managerial positions. In the process, the new manager must also shift his or her focus from an almost exclusively present orientation to a perspective that looks more intently at the future.

Patient/Client Classification Analysis

Patient classification systems are used to categorize patients according to the severity of their illness or the acuteness of their need for nursing care and, in the more sophisticated systems, to predict what level of care is needed (i.e., must the care be provided exclusively by a registered nurse or may some part of the care be provided by another level of staff?). Staff members who see classification systems as financial instruments—which they are, in part—rather than as workload management/ balance tools, sometimes questions the believability of such systems.

Interviewing/Selection Process

The employee selection process includes several elements.

Interviews

Here is a typical interview plan:

1. Greet the interviewee and state the purpose of the interview.
2. Discuss unchangeable aspects of the job, to see if the applicant can meet them.
3. Discuss areas of incomplete information on the application.
4. Describe the job, the department, the organization.
5. Ask a set of structured questions.
6. Encourage the applicant to ask questions and make comments.
7. Tell applicant when to expect a decision and how s/he will be informed of the decision.
8. Thank the applicant for coming in and showing an interest in the job.
9. Evaluate the applicant's suitability for the job immediately after the interview.
10. Complete the interview summary.

Various interviewing methods may be used. The most common methods are as follows.

Structured Interview

For most selection purposes, a structured interview works best, particularly when more than one interviewer is involved. Interviewer judgments are more likely to be

3

consistent when the interviewers use the same approach. Listing the areas to be covered and letting the interviewer determine the order and wording of the questions may accomplish this. Alternatively, a more highly structured approach may be used in which there is a detailed form listing specific questions to be asked with space provided for the answers.

With a structured approach, two or more interviewers will elicit the same information from an applicant, and one interviewer will get approximately the same type of information from two or more candidates for a particular job, thus making comparison easier. One drawback is the lack of flexibility, with the chance that important information about the candidate may not come forth.

Unstructured or Discussion Interview

This approach makes use of nondirective techniques. The result is usually more information about the applicant's opinions and reactions, though not necessarily about characteristics related to anticipated job performance.

Multiple or Group Interview (two options)

1. Several different people interview the applicant, either at separate times, or in a group situation where a panel of interviewers asks questions in turn. This technique is used more often with higher management employees than with frontline staff.
2. The group oral-performance test in which a group of applicants react with each other rather than with the interviewer. Each applicant's behavior can be rated in terms of the effect on the other members of the group. This technique is more often used when deciding to promote current employees rather than in the selection of new employees.

Other activities pertinent to the hiring process include:

- Reference checks. It is important to verify the accuracy of the information included on the candidate's application, even though there are constraints regarding type and depth of information one can obtain from a standard reference check.
- Verification of credentials.
- Testing as required for the particular position (e.g., performance, cognitive, or personality tests) and/or drug testing if required as a matter of institutional policy.
- Physical examination.

The techniques used to recruit and hire employees must be reliable and valid. Reliability refers to the consistency of the hiring process over time. Validity refers to the accuracy of the selection methods (i.e., are the techniques used related to the job for which the applicant is being considered?).

Once placed in a position, a new employee must have the benefit of a well-planned orientation that includes aspects of socialization to the work environment as well as the acquisition of knowledge and skill needed to successfully perform the job.

3

STAFF DEVELOPMENT

Staff-development activities help assure that employees maintain competence and gain new skill and knowledge needed to stay abreast of changes in practice. In earlier times, knowledge was acquired by one generation in order to pass it on to the next generation. Those times are long gone! The body of knowledge in the field of health care is changing constantly and accelerating exponentially. Lifelong learning is not an option: it is a necessity.

ANA's *Scope and Standards of Practice for Nursing Professional Development* (ANA, 2000) provides a framework for the practice of those engaged in staff education and development, as well as for those who administratively support such activities within their institutions.

Standards of Practice for Nursing Staff Development

- **Standard 1. Assessment**
  The nursing professional development educator collects pertinent information related to potential educational needs of the nurse.

- **Standard 2. Diagnosis: Analysis to Determine Target Audience and Learner Needs**
  The nursing professional development educator analyzes the assessment data to determine the target audience and the learner needs.

- **Standard 3. Identification of Educational Outcomes**
  The nursing professional development educator identifies the general purpose and educational objectives for each learning activity.

- **Standard 4. Planning**
  The nursing professional development educator identifies and collaborates with content experts to develop activities to facilitate learners' achievement of the educational objectives.

- **Standard 5. Implementation**
  The nursing professional development educator ensures that the planned educational activities are implemented.

- **Standard 6. Evaluation**
  The nursing professional development educator conducts a comprehensive evaluation of the educational activity.

3

Standards of Professional Performance for Nursing Professional Development

- **Standard 1. Quality of Nursing Professional Development Practice**
  The nursing professional development educator systematically evaluates the quality and effectiveness of nursing professional development practice.

- **Standard 2. Performance Appraisal**
  The nursing professional development educator evaluates his or her own nursing practice in relation to professional practice standards, relevant statutes and regulations, and maintenance of continuing professional nursing competence.

- **Standard 3. Education**
  The nursing professional development educator acquires and maintains current knowledge and competency in nursing professional development practice.

- **Standard 4. Collegiality**
  The nursing professional development educator interacts with, and contributes to the professional development of, peers and other health care providers as colleagues.

- **Standard 5. Ethics**
  The nursing professional development educator's decisions and actions are based on ethical principles.

- **Standard 6. Collaboration**
  The nursing professional development educator collaborates with others in the practice of nursing professional development at the institutional, local, regional, state, national, or international levels.

- **Standard 7. Research**
  The nursing professional development educator participates in and uses evidence-based research to identify strategies for improving professional development activities, nursing practice, and patient outcomes.

- **Standard 8. Management and Resource Utilization**
  The nursing professional development educator considers factors related to safety, effectiveness and cost in planning, delivering, and managing nursing professional development activities.

- **Standard 9. Leadership**
  The nursing professional development educator practices in a manner that provides leadership to the work setting as well as the profession (ANA, 2000).

Needs Assessment

The educational needs assessment should be tied to organizational goals. Specifically, what do employees need to learn or do that is not already part of their practice in order to more efficiently and effectively meet the goals of the organization? Education itself is not the purpose; rather, the educational process is geared toward organizational intent. Such an approach allows better use of whatever educational resources the organization has at its disposal.

Teaching/Learning Principles

The principles of adult learning hold that adults are self-directed, bring with them a wealth of experience upon which to build, must be ready to learn, and learn most effectively when learning is related to the problems at hand.

Learning occurs in three domains: cognitive, affective, and psychomotor. Each domain presents a hierarchy of acquisition. For example, cognition is concerned with intellectual behaviors. The simplest behavior is that of knowledge acquisition in which the person is able to acquire and recall new information. Increasingly sophisticated cognitive elements are comprehension (understand meaning), analysis (distinguish importance of various messages), synthesis (recognize and act), and evaluation (judge significance).

Five levels also are identified in the affective domains: receiving (attend to, listen), responding (participate, react), valuing (assigning worth), organizing (categorizing according to one's value system), and characterizing (acting/responding consistent with values).

In the psychomotor domain, the following hierarchy prevails: perception (awareness), set (physical, mental, and emotional readiness to act), guided response (imitate; perform under the direction of another), mechanism (higher order skill; can put things together and perform more complex tasks), complex overt response (accurately and without hesitation performs complex activities), adaptation (ability to change action according to the situation at hand), and origination (ability to create new movement patterns).

Effective learning depends on three conditions: readiness, ability, and environment. The ability to learn depends on the alignment of these conditions. Identification of the client's preferred learning style is implied here.

Orientation

Orientation programs are designed to familiarize and socialize new staff members to the environment and culture in which they will practice. Planned, structured orientation programs are a mainstay in most organizations, whether for staff new to the facility or new to a particular department. There is no magic formula with

3

regard to the duration of orientation programs. Achievement of orientation objectives, more than time, should ideally drive the length of the orientation. While this approach works in theory, in practice it is not always practical. In general, newly graduated nurses receive a longer orientation than their more seasoned colleagues.

Orientation programs are usually conducted under the auspices of the human resources or educational services departments or units. However, a successful orientation is a shared responsibility with collaboration among the key players critical to achievement of the intended outcome—staff development personnel, the manager, and the new employee.

Inservice Training

Inservice training refers to needs-based training, conducted to fill an identified gap in the employee's skills or knowledge needed to perform effectively in her/his current job. Inservice training is generally linked directly to the practice expectations noted in the employee's job description. Inservice training may be conducted on the job, via computer, via other modes of distance learning, or in a classroom setting. The training is usually brief, practical, and directive; for example, the introduction of a new central line dressing procedure or a change in the safety needle product because of a switch from one vendor to another.

Continuing Education and Professional Development

The rate of change in health care continues to accelerate. Knowledge is obsolete in a matter of months or within a few years at most. The need to remain current in one's professional practice is the responsibility of each clinician. Staff development programs abound. Most are provided by reputable vendors (companies or individuals) or are offered "in-house" to meet the needs of staff members and to help them grow professionally. In contrast to inservice training, continuing education programs are of greater depth, help the learner acquire new knowledge, perhaps in a new or expanded field, and are most often constructed and facilitated by respected experts in a particular field. Continuing education programs may be offered as distance learning programs, seminars, workshops, collegiate or certificate programs, or independent study.

Mentoring, Precepting, and Coaching

Mentors, preceptors, and coaches—what are the differences and are the differences of significance? A mentor is defined as an experienced person who guides and supports the neophyte as s/he gains the needed experience to succeed in the job. The mentor relationship is reciprocal and is generally thought to last for a period of months or, in some cases, even years. Mentor relationships may be structured or unstructured.

A preceptor is one who assumes responsibility for orienting students or new nurses to a given unit or service. The relationship is purposeful, structured, and of relatively short duration. Preceptors themselves generally receive educational preparation for the role and are most often nurses with known clinical expertise and an ability to help new staff members succeed in the assumption of their roles.

A coach is one who helps staff on a day-to-day basis to improve their overall performance. Managers often fill the role of coach. Many do so without benefit of learning interventions designed to prepare them to serve as coaches for their staff.

Competence

According to Benner (1984), competence develops when the nurse begins to see his or her actions in terms of long-range goals or plans about which he or she is consciously aware. The conscious, deliberate planning that is characteristic of this skill level helps achieve efficiency and organization. The competent nurse has a feeling of mastery and the ability to cope with and manage the many contingencies of clinical nursing.

Learning activities linked to the development of competence take into consideration three dimensions of mastery: interpersonal relationships, critical thinking, and clinical practice.

MANAGEMENT ISSUES

Motivation

The extent to which one person can motivate another is a matter for debate. Some theorists maintain that motivation rests entirely with the individual who must act or change in some way, consistent with her/his value system. Others suggest that motivation can be external; that is, a person's behavior can change in response to external factors, for example, to a manager's encouragement or to a perceived reward for changing the way one acts or behaves.

Regardless of how "motivating" a manager might be, a word of caution is in order. If the person who is the object of the manager's attention has neither the ability nor the resources to change, change will not occur and attempts to motivate change will be met with frustration.

Perhaps it is more important for managers who wish to motivate their employees to establish the environment that will allow change to happen and to assure that the employees have the needed resources to embrace change within themselves and within the workplace.

3

Communication

Communication is the exchange of thoughts, messages, or information, by speech, signals, writing, or behavior. Communication implies that there is mutual understanding of the message sent and the message received. Much of what is assumed to be communication is merely information delivery. Whether or not the intent of the communication is understood and accepted is unknown.

Exquisite communication skills are perhaps the manager's most valuable assets. And active listening may be the crowning achievement! As alternatives to face-to-face communication become the norm (e.g., e-mail and voicemail), the likelihood of miscommunication increases significantly.

Delegation

Delegation is the assignment of new or additional responsibilities to a subordinate. The person to whom the task (function, activity, or decision) is delegated accepts the authority and responsibility for completion of the assignment. The subordinate is expected to report to the manager regarding how effectively s/he was able to complete the assigned task. Delegation, particularly of day-to-day, in-the-moment tasks, is fundamental to managerial effectiveness because it allows the manager to focus on issues of greater long-term significance to the health of the enterprise.

In the delegation process, managers are advised to keep in mind three key concepts: responsibility, authority, and accountability. Responsibility implies an obligation to complete a task. Accountability means accepting ownership for the results or lack thereof. Responsibility is transferred; accountability is shared. Authority is the right to act. This means that the manager (delegator) has empowered the subordinate (delegatee) to accomplish the task. Managers sometimes fall into a trap of their own making: they delegate responsibility without giving authority. This sets up the subordinate for failure with a resultant decrease in efficiency and productivity.

Effective delegation has several benefits:

- The delegator is able to devote more time to tasks that cannot be delegated;
- The delegatee develops new skills and abilities;
- Delegation facilitates upward mobility for the delegatee;
- It builds self-esteem and confidence;
- It improves morale; fosters a sense of pride in abilities;
- It allows individuals to appreciate the roles and responsibilities of others;
- The organization's bottom line may improve.

Steps in the delegation process include:

- Define the task;
- Determine who will or is able to perform the task;
- Describe expectations;
- Come to agreement;
- Monitor results and provide feedback.

Relationships

Interpersonal

Interpersonal communication describes the exchange of information and meaning between two or more people through verbal and nonverbal interplay in a face-to-face encounter. Interpersonal communication is often informal and its success (or failure) depends on the existence of established relationships.

Professional

Professional or public communication implies interaction with large groups of people. The message sender must be acutely aware of the intent and content of the message and of the style used to convey the message. Posture, body movement, timing, and tone of voice all play a role in successful professional communication.

Team Building

The abilities to express one's ideas clearly and decisively, to listen attentively and respectfully, and to invite a range of opinions are among the communication skills that help managers build team cohesiveness through communication.

Cultural Considerations

Cultural aspects of communication also deserve attention, particularly as members of the workforce and the patient populations cared for in the health care system become increasingly diverse. While bilingual or multilingual skills are of great value in today's workplace, of equal importance is an understanding of the beliefs, values, and practices of the groups served. And, while cultural generalizations may be helpful, stereotyping is not. Any and all assumptions related to cultural practices or beliefs should be verified before they are acted on.

Conflict and Conflict Resolution

Conflict occurs naturally in and among groups and individuals; conflict is inevitable and is a condition essential to change. Conflict may be interpersonal (within oneself), interpersonal (between the self and another person), intragroup (among members of a particular group), or intergroup (among members of two or more groups). Other types of conflict include competitive conflict and disruptive or destructive conflict. In both instances, the desired outcome is to overcome one's opponent, that is, to "win."

Conflict management occupies a significant portion of the manager's work. Some suggest that at least one quarter of the manager's time is spent in conflict management activities. The challenge for the manager is, of course, to help her/his subordinates reach a win-win outcome in which the parties to the conflict each believe they have come away from the encounter with a sense of resolution. Win-win strategies include: focusing on goals, not personalities; meeting the needs of both parties, equally if at all possible; and building consensus. Achieving "win-win" is much easier in the abstract than in the workplace setting. Nonetheless, it is a worthwhile goal.

Decision Making

Managerial decisions fall into a number of categories. Routine decisions are those involving such things as policies and procedures and the day-to-day business of the department. Such decisions are generally within the realm of first-line managers. Adaptive decisions are more complex and arise in the presence of problems that are out of the ordinary and not fully understood. The manager may apply or adapt a decision-making process used previously to the current situation. Innovative decisions are called for when the problems are unusual, unclear, and have no precedent.

The conditions under which managers must make decisions vary. Decisions may be made under certainty (conditions and alternatives are known), under risk (only some of the conditions are known and their relative probability can be determined), or under uncertainty (risks, alternatives and/or consequences are unknown). In reality, most major decisions are made under conditions of risk or uncertainty.

Steps in the decision-making process include:

- Identifying and diagnosing the problem
- Generating alternative solutions
- Evaluating alternatives
- Choosing the decision
- Implementing the decision
- Evaluating the decision

Recognition

Well-executed reward and recognition programs contribute to overall employee satisfaction. Recognition can be intangible; for example, employee-of-the month designation, letters of commendation, public acknowledgement of the contributions of individuals or groups. Alternatively, it may be tangible, such as bonuses, salary increases, vacation trips, and various types of gifts.

Recognition of individuals is most valued when it comes from one's immediate supervisor, followed closely by recognition from one's peers and one's customers or subordinates. To be meaningful, recognition must be honest and sincere; otherwise, it is perceived as manipulative and pointless.

Job Satisfaction

Job satisfaction is related to the quality of work life (QWL) and companies now devote time and resources to improving working conditions in a number of dimensions: compensation that is fair and adequate; a physical environment that is safe and healthy; jobs that are appropriately challenging and rewarding in and of themselves; opportunities for personal and professional growth; a social environment that is harmonious; a work role that allows for balance in other dimensions of one's life; and affiliation with a socially conscious organization.

A psychological contract exists between employees and employers. The contract is composed of a set of perceptions about what employees owe their employers and what employers owe their employees. When either party believes the contract has been "violated," conflict may arise, then escalate or diminish depending on how well or quickly equilibrium is restored.

Group Dynamics

Social scientists have identified predictable stages of group development. The first stage is known as **forming**. Individuals come together and form a defined cluster. People are cautious in their communication with one another; they are still relative strangers and rely on a leader to define and direct their activities.

As the group proceeds through the maturation process, it arrives at the second stage known as **storming**. In this stage, members of the group compete for position, power, and status; informal leaders may emerge. The (formal) leader helps the group identify and work through conflict.

The third stage of group formation is called **norming**. Here the rules for working collaboratively are made explicit; structure, roles, and relationships are clarified. The leader's role is to advance relationship building.

As the group matures, it enters the **performing** stage: it is in this mode that the work of the group is most effectively carried out. The energy of the group is focused on achieving its goals in a collaborative atmosphere. The leader's role is to provide feedback on the work that the group is accomplishing, redirect group energy when necessary, and further cultivate interpersonal relationships.

A number of experts suggest that the group formation process, and thus the productivity of the group, can be accelerated under the guidance of a skillful facilitator or in the face of actual or fabricated crisis.

Negotiation

Negotiation can be thought of as a formal process; for example, the negotiations that take place at the time of contract deliberations between unions and management. Negotiation can also be thought of as a political process. The implication here is that the negotiation process is a "power play" among individuals who compete to "win" but generally compromise in the end.

3

Interest-based negotiation is a somewhat newer concept, the principles of which were outlined by Fisher and Ury in *Getting to Yes* (1991). Bizony (1999) has distilled the principles listed below from Fisher and Ury's work on the Harvard Negotiation Project; their value has been convincingly promulgated through the years:

- Treat people as equals, resolve issues on their merits.
- Define the issue so that the definition is acceptable to all parties.
- Focus on interests, not on conclusions or positions.
- Develop options that may meet the interests of both parties.
- Apply objective standards to resolve conflicting Interests.

Discipline

Disciplinary action occurs when rules are broken. Organizations should have a fair and well-organized disciplinary process in place for the protection of all parties involved. Managers are advised to consult with their human resources department when they find it necessary to discipline employees. In this way, they assure that the rights of the employee and those of the organization are protected. Policies should provide for progressive discipline, leading, if necessary, to termination without recrimination.

Depending on the severity of the infraction, the disciplinary process may provide for immediate dismissal or for investigatory suspension with or without pay. While managers may themselves be distressed when faced with a situation that requires discipline, it is helpful for them to keep in mind the reason for the disciplinary action. The disciplinary process should be thought of not as punishment but as an opportunity to teach and encourage the person or persons involved in the infraction.

Most organizations subscribe to a progressive discipline process in which counseling and intervention are cumulative. In a union environment, disciplinary action may be "grieved" consistent with the grievance process outlined in the labor contract. The grievance process is seen as a means to give workers a voice in what goes on during contract negotiation and administration.

Employee Assistance Programs

Employee assistance programs (EAPs) may be in-house or outsourced. EAPs exist to help organizations address productivity issues and to help employees identify and resolve personal concerns such as family, financial, health, legal, alcohol and/or drug, and stress issues that interfere with their ability to function effectively in the job. EAP professionals are skilled counselors and are ethically obligated to remain neutral in their counsel.

Stress Management

Job stress disrupts psychological and/or physiological balance. It takes a toll at the personal, organizational, and societal level and is manifest in the phenomenon known as "burnout."

Stress reduction techniques can be learned and adapted to any work setting. Their intent is to improve physical and mental well-being and to enable a person to identify and cope more successfully with stressors. There is no magic to the stress management techniques listed here; all are in the realm of common sense. Yet they are practiced all too infrequently to the detriment of many, including managers and executives in "high pressure" positions whose job demands seems to be ever increasing.

- Habituation — "routinize" tasks whenever possible; predictability means less chance of surprise; establishing routines conserves energy.
- Time block — calendar time for predictable tasks and remain on task during the blocked time. If necessary, block time for such ephemeral activities as thinking, reflecting, or meditating. These are not "time wasters," they are tasks critical to the manager's success in her/his position and in life.
- Time management — learning to say "no" may be the best time management technique for the busy manager! Numerous time management techniques exist; the literature and workshop offerings are replete with suggestions. It is important to remember that the use of a "Palm Pilot' or a "Daytimer" is not synonymous with time management. Taking the time to evaluate how one spends her/his time on the job is often a most revealing exercise and inevitably points to opportunities for change.
- Environmental modification — changing one's physical or social environment may help reduce stress. Creating a quiet place in which to work, eliminating non-essential committee work, using sound, scent, color, and texture to modify one's environment are helpful techniques.
- Regular exercise, proper diet and nutrition, rest, incorporation of relaxation techniques into day-to-day living, development of support systems, and crisis intervention plans are practical activities that reduced stress in any setting.

It is interesting that nurses are among the first to promote stress management techniques for their clients/patients but are also among the most reluctant to adopt these same techniques in their own lives.

Personnel Policies and Procedures

The availability of up-to-date, legally sound personnel policies is essential to managers and executives. Some organizations now maintain their personnel manuals in an on-line format, making them instantaneously available to managers at the time they are needed.

3

Personnel policies govern such crucial management functions as recruitment, conducting interviews, hiring, rewards and discipline, counseling, resignation and discharge, transfers, compensation, timekeeping, compliance with labor laws, compliance with contracts (in a union environment), orientation, and evaluation/assessment.

Most organizations conduct episodic workshops for managers to help them remain abreast of the latest regulations governing the workplace from a personnel perspective.

Performance Appraisal

The performance appraisal is often thought of an as event rather than as an ongoing process. Despite the admonition that "there should be no surprises" when the manager and the staff member sit down together to review the employee's performance, this caution rarely holds. Performance appraisals serve an administrative purpose in that they are used for making promotion, salary, or, in some cases, layoff decisions. They also have a developmental purpose in that the assessment can be used to identify training needs, career planning, leadership potential, and so forth.

Performance appraisals can occur in a variety of ways. Here are a few of them:

Peer Review

Peer review occurs when nurses have determined the standards and criteria that constitute quality care and judge their practice against the standards. Standards are evidence based and are representative of the values of the profession. Advance practice nurses in particular engage in the peer review process and may be required to do so from a regulatory standpoint.

Management by Objectives

Results-oriented evaluations measure employee performance relative to goals or targets achieved or objectives attained (management by objectives). This type of performance appraisal is often used for those in managerial and administrative roles.

Criteria-Based Objectives

Criteria-based evaluations are those that measure or assess the employee's performance in relation to well-defined requirements of the job. Employees either meet or do not meet the standards established for a particular position.

Self-Evaluation

Self-evaluation is defined by the term itself. Employees are often asked to engage in self-evaluation as part of the overall appraisal process. The employee and his/her manager then compare notes and negotiate a mutually acceptable final appraisal.

Regardless of the appraisal process used, managers are advised to keep the following guidelines in mind:

- Take legal considerations into account.
- Relate performance standards to job analysis (they should match).
- Communicate standards to staff (no surprises).
- Evaluate employee practice on performance-related behaviors, not on global measures.
- Document the process.
- Use more than one rater whenever possible (for example, the 360° process).
- Assure that an appeal process is in place.

Absenteeism

A study conducted in 2000 by the Gale Group found that personal illness (21%), family issues (21%), and personal needs (20%) accounted for nearly two-thirds of unscheduled absences from work. Stress (19%) and an entitlement mentality (19%) were not far behind. According to some analysts, there has been more than a 300% increase in stress-related absenteeism since 1995. The number of hours Americans are working, compared with their counterparts in other industrial nations, may account in part for the increase in stress-related absenteeism.

Work-life programs can be effective in controlling absenteeism, though many companies have been slow to implement such initiatives. Work-life programs with the most appeal include childcare referral, leave for school functions, flexible scheduling, emergency childcare, compressed workweek, and on-site childcare. Of those ranked highest by employees only flexible scheduling was a "match" among the programs offered by employers, with over half reporting that they had flexible-hour arrangements in place.

Work-life programs offered by a given company must be consonant with the organization's purpose and with employee demographics. There is no "one size fits all" work-life program. However, there is general agreement that investments in well-planned work-life initiatives are less costly than ever-increasing absenteeism.

Initiatives to reduce absence include paid time off (provides employees with a bank of hours to be used for various purposes instead of separate accounts for sick, vacation, and personal time) and no-fault systems, which limit the number of unscheduled absences allowed, regardless of circumstances, and take specific disciplinary actions if that number is exceeded.

Job Enrichment

Various techniques are available to increase the intrinsic satisfaction with one's job. Job **rotation** implies that boredom can be reduced and satisfaction increased if the employee can periodically move from one job to another, or from one task to another within a job, provided s/he has the capacity to perform the tasks associated with each rotation.

3

Job **enlargement** means that the employee is given additional tasks to do, not merely rotated from task to task. Job **enrichment** implies that the employee is given higher levels of responsibility or that the job itself is redesigned or restructured. Of the three approaches, job enrichment is seen as the most satisfying to the employee.

Within the field of nursing, a word of caution is in order. Scope of practice issues must be considered when and if any of the above approaches are suggested. In addition, in a union environment, the techniques described may not be acceptable or may be achieved only through negotiation.

Management Style

Managerial or leadership style is traditionally described in these terms, particularly as they relate to the manager's decision-making style: participative, democratic, autocratic, or laissez-faire. The participative manager involves his/her employees in the decision-making process; the democratic manager solicits input from his/her subordinates; the autocratic manager makes decisions on her own and announces them to others; and the laissez-faire manager decides by not deciding.

Few managers subscribe exclusively to one model and are more likely to be described as having a contingency style, which means they adjust their approach to the needs and demands of the situation. Managers can and do identify their preferred leadership style, but this is generally done as a developmental task that allows them to strengthen desirable skills required in their jobs.

Supervision and Delegation

Delegation pertains to the concepts of accountability, responsibility, and authority. Delegation is the reciprocal process in which responsibility and authority for a given function is transferred to another individual who accepts the authority and responsibility. Responsibility implies an obligation to carry out a task; accountability means accepting ownership for the results or lack of results. In delegation, responsibility is transferred; however, accountability is shared. Authority is the right to act.

It is important for nurses/nurse managers to understand their legal responsibilities when delegating tasks to and supervising other staff members. The nurse is liable for the reasonable exercise of his/her delegation and supervision activities. This means s/he must be aware of the knowledge, skills, competencies, and scope of practice of staff members when delegating tasks and is obligated to supervise effectively. It does not mean the registered nurse is responsible for the tasks performed by others. That responsibility rests with the staff member to whom the task was delegated.

CHAPTER 4

Ethics

PROFESSIONAL ETHICS

Professions are defined, in part, by the ethics that govern their practice. While nursing has long been recognized for its commitment to high ethical standards, that commitment was further endorsed in 1990 with the establishment of the Center for Ethics and Human Rights under the aegis of the American Nurses Association (ANA). The center is "committed to addressing the complex ethical and human rights issues confronting nurses and designing activities and programs to increase the ethical competence and human rights sensitivity of nurses." The rich library of resources available through the center is found at this Web address: **www. nursingworld.org/ethics/.**

Values Clarification

Cultural Diversity

The diverse beliefs and value systems that clients/patients, staff, and practitioners bring with them to the health care environment speak to the need for managers to expand their knowledge of diversity from an ethical as well as from a business perspective.

Dimensions of diversity include age, gender, sexual orientation, ability/disability, ethnicity, socioeconomic status, education, origin, and so forth. The Code of Ethics that governs the practice of nursing compels managers to practice "with compassion and respect for the inherent dignity, worth and uniqueness of every individual, unrestricted by considerations of social or economic status, personal attributes or the nature of health problems."

The manager is challenged to integrate and interpret disparate points of view among and within the staff he/she manages as well as among and between the client groups served and the staff who serve them. For example, there may be no words in "high context" languages to compare with the "low context" English terminology used to explain certain procedures or interventions. Imagine attempting to explain "do not resuscitate" to someone who has no reference point for the concept of "resuscitation."

Professional Integrity

Integrity is defined as strict adherence to a code of conduct that is above reproach. The hallmarks of a profession are noted here:

- An extended education (body of knowledge) that sets its members apart;
- A theoretical body of knowledge leading to defined skills, abilities, and norms;
- Provision of a specific practice (of value to society and for which society cannot provide independent of the profession);
- Autonomy in decision making and practice;
- The existence of a code of ethics that governs the practice of the members of the profession.

Managers have an ongoing opportunity to exemplify professional integrity in their work and to influence the practice of their subordinates by example.

Code for Nurses

The abbreviated version of the most recently updated Code of Ethics for Nurses is presented here. The full *Code for Nurses with Interpretive Statements* monograph is available through ANA. Further information about obtaining the booklet can be found on the *Nursing World* Web site identified on page 91.

Code of Ethics for Nurses

- The nurse, in all professional relationships, practices with compassion and respect for the inherent dignity, worth and uniqueness of every individual, unrestricted by considerations of social or economic status, personal attributes or the nature of health problems.
- The nurse's primary commitment is to the patient, whether an individual, family group or community.
- The nurse promotes, advocates for and strives to protect the health, safety and rights of the patient.
- The nurse is responsible and accountable for individual nursing practice and determines the appropriate delegation of tasks consistent with the nurse's obligation to provide optimum patient care.
- The nurse owes the same duties to self as to others, including the responsibility to preserve integrity and safety, to maintain competence and to continue personal and professional growth.
- The nurse participates in establishing, maintaining and improving health care environments and conditions of employment conducive to the provision of quality health care and consistent with the values of the profession through individual and collective action.

4

- The nurse participates in the advancement of the profession through contributions to practice, education, administration and knowledge development.
- The nurse collaborates with other health professionals and the public in promoting community, national and international efforts to meet health needs.
- The profession of nursing, as represented by associations and their members, is responsible for articulating nursing values, for maintaining the integrity if the profession and its practice and for shaping social policy. (© September 2001, American Nurses Association. Reprinted with permission.)

Confidentiality

The absolute need to maintain confidentiality in practice is a tenet so dear that its violation may, under certain circumstances, result in immediate termination of employment. With the implementation of HIPAA (Health Insurance Portability and Accountability Act of 1996), civil and criminal penalties can be levied when legal requirements regarding confidentiality are ignored or violated.

Refusal of Assignment

Staff members retain the right to refuse an assignment based on their own deeply held beliefs. This situation usually arises in the presence of termination of pregnancy cases or of withdrawal of life support. In the coming years, managers and administrators should anticipate the potential dilemmas related to genetic engineering and its possible impact on the acceptance or refusal of assignments by staff members.

Ethical Theories

Two major theoretical perspectives form the foundation for dialogue about ethical issues pertinent to health care: the deontological approach and the teleological approach. Deontology holds that an act is good unto itself. It is sometimes described as the theory rooted in "rules." It holds that certain rules must be followed or actions taken regardless of the consequences. For example, if the belief is that the truth must always be told, there is no reason to not tell the truth, under any circumstance.

On the other hand, teleological theorists hold that the end or purpose of an action determines its rightness or wrongness. Utilitarianism is the prime example of the teleological belief system. Utility holds that "the greatest good for the greatest number" is the desired end point and that the relative "right" or "wrong" of acts is less important that the consequence of those acts. For example, it may be morally acceptable for a mother to steal a loaf of bread to feed her family if the only other option open to her is their starvation.

4

Ethical Principles

Here, briefly described, are the major ethical principles that guide those in the field of health care:

- **Respect for individuals.** Human beings are autonomous; that is they have the capacity for rational action and moral choice and have a value unto themselves. Their choices and judgment should be respected and should not be interfered with unless they are clearly harmful to others. The degree of **autonomy** varies to some degree according to the person's capacity for decision making and choice on his/her own behalf. For example, the infant has the potential for autonomy, but not yet the capacity. In addition to autonomy, **veracity** (truth-telling), **confidentiality**, and the concept of **informed consent** are derived from the principle of respect for individuals.
- **Beneficence** holds that first, one has an obligation to do no harm, and second, one has an obligation to promote good. The principle of beneficence is basic to medicine. The extent to which beneficence and autonomy are competing values rests at the heart of discourse about ethical dilemmas. For example, if the physician believes that, with another round of aggressive radiation, she may "buy more time" for the patient, but the patient, who is aware and fully informed, chooses to forgo the radiation with the knowledge that his decision will certainly hasten death, then the patient's desire for autonomy and the physician's commitment to beneficence may be in conflict.
- **Justice** as an ethical principle means "that which is fair or that which is deserved." The concept of "rights" is associated with justice, as is the notion of obligation. The ethical issues surrounding allocation of resources are often seen as promoting or neglecting the principle of justice. For example, a patient with a predictably terminal illness hears about a costly experimental treatment for his disease, wants to have the treatment, and asks his health maintenance organization (HMO) to assume the cost of the treatment. The HMO refuses because the action would be precedent setting and the principle of justice held by the organization—the "most good for the most people"—would be vaulted. Utilitarian justice guides the decision in this case.

Ethical Dilemmas

An ethical dilemma exists in the presence of competing values in which the community, as well as the individuals involved, has a vested interest. Health care institutions have formalized the existence of multidisciplinary ethics committees as advisory bodies to help sort through the dilemmas faced by patients, their caregivers, and their families.

A systematic approach to the identification and meaning of the ethical issues is suggested. One such approach is outlined by those involved in the Ethics in Medicine Division of the University of Washington's School of Medicine. The recommended "ethics workup" includes a review of medical indications, patient preferences, quality of life, and contextual issues. The workup describes "what is." Then, the deliberation moves to the next phase and involves questions such as these:

- What is at issue?
- Where is the conflict?
- What is this case about? Is it similar to other cases encountered? What is known about them?
- Is there precedent? Is there a paradigm case (e.g., Quinlan, Cruzan)?
- Who is involved and what roles do they play?

Cultural values may be at the center of ethical dilemmas. For example, the commitment to honor end-of-life care preferences has been codified and patients are now routinely asked about the availability of an advance directive for health care or living will. If the patient's background is such that death is a taboo subject, perhaps because of a belief system that holds "to speak of death invites him in the door," then discussions about life support or the withdrawal of life-support interventions may be inappropriate from the standpoint of the family/patient, but greatly desired by the health care team.

ETHICS AND HUMAN VALUES

Patient/Client Rights

The concept of patient rights has taken on new importance in recent years. In 1973, the American Hospital Association published a list of patient rights that has been used as issued or in slightly edited versions since that time. Patients are generally provided with a copy of their rights upon entry into the acute care setting; similar rights are accorded those in long-term care, rehabilitation care, and so forth. State law may mandate such provision. A patient's rights include:

- The right to considerate and respectful care.
- The right to get complete, up-to-date information about his diagnosis, treatment, and prognosis (expected outcome) from his physician in terms the patient can reasonably be expected to understand. If it is not medically advisable to give this information to the patient, it should be given to another appropriate person on his behalf. The patient (or the appropriate person) has the right to know by name the physician who is responsible for coordinating the care of the patient.
- The right to get enough information about any proposed treatment or procedure to make an "informed consent"—that is, he should know enough about the expected benefits, possible hazards, and time needed for recovery to decide if he wants that treatment or procedure. This information should come from the patient's doctor and should be provided in every case except in an emergency where delay could harm the patient.

4

- The right to be told about alternatives to the proposed treatment and/or procedure, and the right to know who will be responsible for the treatment and/or procedure.
- The right to refuse treatment to the extent permitted by law, and to be informed of the possible medical consequences of doing so.
- The right to every consideration of his privacy concerning his own medical care program. Case discussion, consultation, examination, and treatment are confidential and should be conducted discreetly. Those not directly involved in his care must have the permission of the patient to be present.
- The right to expect that all communications and records concerning his care should be treated as confidential.
- The right to expect the hospital to make a reasonable response to his request for services. Depending on how urgent the patient's medical problem is, the hospital must evaluate the patient, and then must provide service or referral. If the patient is to be transferred to another facility, he must first receive all the information and an explanation of why a transfer needs to be made. The institution to which the patient is to be transferred must accept the patient before he is transferred. The patient has the right to be informed of any relations the hospital has to any other health care and/or education institutions if the relationship may affect his care.
- The right to know if any of the people treating him have any professional relationships among themselves that might affect his care.
- The right to be told if the hospital plans to engage in any human experimentation that might affect his care or treatment. The patient has the right to refuse to participate in such research projects.
- The right to expect reasonable continuity of care. He has the right to know in advance what appointment times and physicians are available and where they will be. The patient has the right to be informed about what his continuing health care requirements will be after discharge.
- The right to examine and receive an explanation of his bill regardless of whether it's paid by him or another source.
- The right to know what hospital rules and regulations apply to his conduct as a patient.

Advocacy

Advocates are those who stand in for or "plead the cause of" those who cannot speak for themselves. Nurses often described themselves as "patient advocates." However, because nurses are accountable to constituencies whose values are occasionally at odds with one another, the assumption that the nurse will always act as a patient advocate may present a dilemma. When faced with such a quandary, nurses may elect to apply an ethical framework as part of their decision making process. Here is one approach:

- What are the medical/health care issues that present themselves in the situation?
- What are the patient's preferences (to the extent they are known or can be discovered)?
- What is the quality of life for the patient (from her/his perspective, not that of the nurse)?
- What is the context surrounding the situation? What familial, legal, economic, and/or institutional considerations must be taken into consideration as part of the deliberations? (University of Washington, School of Medicine/Ethics in Medicine, **http://depts.washington.edu/bioethx/**).

Advance Directives

The Patient Self-Determination Act, passed in 1990 and enacted in 1991, requires that all individuals receiving medical care must be given written information about their rights under state law to make decisions about their care, including the right to accept or refuse medical or surgical treatment. Individuals must also be given information about their rights to formulate advance directives such as living wills and durable powers of attorney for health care. Patients must be made aware of their rights to make decisions about these issues upon admission (in the case of hospitals or skilled nursing facilities), enrollment (in the case of health maintenance organizations), on first receipt of care (in the case of hospices), or before the patient comes under an agency's care (in the case of home health-personal care agencies).

Nurses have a critical role to play in end-of-life care and the voice of the profession is very much in evidence thanks to initiatives such as the End-of Life Nursing Education Consortium (ELNEC) project. In collaboration with the Robert Wood Johnson Foundation, the American Association of Colleges of Nursing (AACN) began the ELNEC project in 2000. ELNEC is a national education initiative to improve end-of-life care in the United States. The project provides nurse educators with training in end-of-life care so they can teach this essential information to nursing students and practicing nurses.

Organ Donation and Transplants

The number of people on waiting lists for organ transplants far exceeds available organs. At the present time, those whose names are at the top of most lists are people who have become so seriously ill that they need to receive viable organs within a relatively short period of time to forestall inevitable death.

To assure equity in the distribution of scarce organs, a computer data bank has been established. Its intent is to quickly match donors with recipients and to facilitate the delivery of organs in a timely manner in order to increase the probability of successful transplantation.

4

A few of the topical ethical issues surrounding organ donation include the following:

- Do people have the "right" to bypass the organ donor system and petition for organs via the Internet?
- If the person is successful in procuring an organ, is the health care system under any obligation to perform the transplant?
- Is it acceptable to "purchase" organs or to offer some type of financial recompense for donated organs?
- Should "healthier" transplant candidates be placed at the top of the waiting list in preference to the very ill so that the donated organs will "last longer"?
- Do the uninsured poor have the same right to organs as those with insurance? If the answer is yes, who assumes financial risk for the procedure and for follow-up care?
- Do people wanting experimental transplant procedures have the right to expect their managed care insurer to pay for the procedure contrary to the terms of the agreement with the carrier?
- Rather than requesting permission to proceed with organ removal in the face of an inevitable outcome of death, should the medical community assume consent and automatically harvest much needed organs?

Soon ethical dilemmas related to genetics, including DNA manipulation and organ cloning, will overshadow the ethical quandaries posed by organ donation and transplantation.

Resource Utilization

Ethical concerns surround the allocation of scarce resources in the field of health care. Perhaps the most cogent question is the one that is seldom asked, that is: If waste were to be removed from the system, would resources still be scarce? While ethicists and philosophers debate the question around the theme of "justice," those on the frontline of the delivery system make daily decisions that compel them to say no to some objective good, so that they can say yes to a competing need.

At least one health care system in the United States has taken ethical discourse beyond that which ponders case-by-case dilemmas at the bedside and brought the discussion into the boardroom where top-level decision makers have agreed to add an ethical filter to their resource allocation deliberations. The degree to which this approach will be adopted more widely is unknown at this time.

4

CHAPTER 5

Legal and Regulatory Issues

FEDERAL AND STATE

Federal Laws and Regulations

Occupational Safety and Health Administration (OSHA)

OSHA is a broadly written piece of legislation that covers any employer engaged in a business affecting commerce, requiring that employer to "furnish to each of his employees a place of employment which is free from recognized hazards that are causing, or are likely to cause death or serious physical harm." This federal legislation was modeled after the California (Cal-OSHA) program that was in effect before the establishment of the federal plan in 1970.

OSHA is authorized to conduct workplace inspections on every business covered by the act. Obviously, it is impossible for the Department of Labor, the federal department in which the OSHA resides, to inspect every entity covered by the law. Thus, OSHA inspections are generally conducted at the request of the employer (to verify potentially unsafe conditions) or in response to a complaint from an employee. According to OSHA, reporting priorities are assessed in this order:

> Top priority are reports of imminent dangers—accidents about to happen; second are fatalities or accidents serious enough to send three or more workers to the hospital. Third are employee complaints. Referrals from other government agencies are fourth. Fifth are targeted inspections—such as the Site Specific Targeting Program, which focuses on employers that report high injury and illness rates, and special emphasis programs that zero in on hazardous work such as trenching or equipment such as mechanical power presses. Follow-up inspections are the final priority.

Since the agency was created in 1971 with the goal of reducing workplace injuries and deaths, "occupational deaths have been cut in half and injuries have declined by 40 percent" (**www.osha.gov**). The Act has been amended a number of times since its inception.

Recordkeeping is required to verify compliance with the act. OSHA forms are supplied to employers for this purpose. With the advent of online technology, the forms are now available through the Internet. About 1.3 million employers with 11 or more employees—20% of the establishments OSHA covers—must keep records of work-related injuries and illnesses. Workplaces in low-hazard industries such as retail, service, finance, insurance, and real estate are exempt from record-keeping requirements. Health care organizations are obviously not among the exempted employers.

There are two major types of laws in the field of occupational health and safety: **compensatory and preventive.** OSHA is an example of preventive law. The well-known compensatory laws that have been enacted are **worker compensation** laws. Under worker compensation, an employee who is injured or becomes ill as a result of a condition on the job is compensated for that injury, including reimbursement of medical and hospital costs, whether or not his own acts caused or contributed to causing the injury.

Omnibus Budget Reconciliation Acts

Congress passed the landmark Consolidated Omnibus Budget Reconciliation Act (COBRA) health benefit provisions in 1986. The law amends the Employee Retirement Income Security Act (ERISA), the Internal Revenue Code, and the Public Health Service Act to provide continuation of group health coverage that otherwise might be terminated.

COBRA contains provisions giving certain former employees, retirees, spouses, former spouses, and dependent children the right to temporary continuation of health coverage at group rates. This coverage, however, is only available when coverage is lost due to certain specific events. Group health coverage for COBRA participants is usually more expensive than health coverage for active employees, since usually the employer pays a part of the premium for active employees while COBRA participants generally pay the entire premium themselves. It is ordinarily less expensive, though, than individual health coverage.

The law generally covers group health plans maintained by employers with 20 or more employees in the prior year. It applies to plans in the private sector and to those sponsored by state and local governments. The law does not, however, apply to plans sponsored by the federal government and certain church-related organizations.

Group health plans sponsored by private sector employers generally are welfare benefit plans governed by ERISA and subject to its requirements for reporting and disclosure, fiduciary standards, and enforcement. ERISA does not establish minimum standards or benefit eligibility for welfare plans or mandate the type or level of benefits offered to plan participants.

The original health continuation provisions were contained in Title X of COBRA, which was signed into law (Public Law 99–272) on April 7, 1986. Provisions of COBRA covering state and local government plans are administered by the Department of Health and Human Services.

There are three elements to qualifying for COBRA benefits. COBRA establishes specific criteria for plans, qualified beneficiaries, and qualifying events.

- **Plan Coverage.** Group health plans for employers with 20 or more employees on more than 50% of its typical business days in the previous calendar year are subject to COBRA. Both full- and part-time employees are counted to determine whether a plan is subject to COBRA. Each part-time employee counts as a fraction of an employee, with the fraction equal to the number of hours that the part-time employee worked divided by the hours an employee must work to be considered full time.

- **Qualified Beneficiaries.** A qualified beneficiary generally is an individual covered by a group health plan on the day before a qualifying event who either is an employee, the employee's spouse, or an employee's dependent child. In certain cases, a retired employee, the retired employee's spouse, and the retired employee's dependent children may be qualified beneficiaries. In addition, any child born to or placed for adoption with a covered employee during the period of COBRA coverage is considered a qualified beneficiary. Agents, independent contractors, and directors who participate in the group health plan may also be qualified beneficiaries.
- **Qualifying Events.** Qualifying events are certain events that would cause an individual to lose health coverage. The type of qualifying event will determine who the qualified beneficiaries are and the amount of time that a plan must offer the health coverage to them under COBRA.

Patient Self-Determination Act (Public Law 101–508)

On December 1, 1991, federal legislation known as the Patient Self-Determination Act (PSDA) took effect in hospitals, skilled nursing faculties, home health agencies, hospice organizations, and health maintenance organizations serving Medicare and Medicaid patients. The PSDA requires these institutions to develop and maintain written policies and procedures to provide written information to adults for whom the institutions provide care. These materials must describe:

- Individuals' rights under the law to make decisions about medical care, including the right to accept or refuse medical and surgical treatment;
- Individuals' rights under state law to dictate advance directives such as living wills or durable powers of attorney for health care and the policies and procedures that the institution has developed to honor these rights. Institutions must specify how the advance directives are to be identified, recorded, and retrieved when needed. The legislation requires institutions to provide educational programs on advance directives for their staff and communities. It prohibits staff from conditioning the provision of care or discriminating against individuals in other ways because they do or do not have advance directives. Hospitals and nursing homes must provide all newly admitted patients with written information detailing these policies and procedures, and home health and hospice agencies must provide information when the individual begins to receive care from the agency

Americans with Disabilities Act

Under the Americans with Disabilities Act (ADA), the term "disability" with respect to an individual has three distinct definitions: 1) a physical or mental impairment that substantially limits one or more of the major life activities; 2) a record of such impairment; or 3) being regarded as having such an impairment. An individual must satisfy at least one of these definitions in order to be considered an individual with a disability for the purposes of this act.

President George Bush signed the ADA into law on July 26, 1990. The act is designed to ensure that otherwise qualified individuals with disabilities enjoy the same employment opportunities enjoyed by non-disabled persons. The Equal Employment Opportunity Commission published its final regulations implementing the equal employment provisions of the ADA on July 26, 1991. The ADA is organized into five separate titles:

- **Title I. Employment** — Prohibits employers from discriminating based on an individual's disabilities and applies to all facets of employment, including application for employment and terms of employment.
- **Title II. Public Services** — Requires public entities employed in public transportation services to provide accessible services to the disabled.
- **Title III. Public Accommodations and Services Operated by Private Entities** — Prohibits discrimination in places of public accommodations provided by private entities, such as lodgings, restaurants, educational facilities, etc.
- **Title IV. Telecommunications Relay Services** — Requires carriers of telephonic services to provide equal communication opportunities to disables persons.
- **Title V. Provisions** — Provides certain miscellaneous provisions, including state immunity, attorney fees, and prohibition against employer retaliation.

Effective dates for Title I and Employment Provisions of Title I which most affect employers:

- For employers with 25 or more employees: July 27, 1992.
- For employers with 15 or more employees: July 27, 1994.

Title I reads: "No covered entity shall discriminate against a qualified individual with a disability because of the disability of such individual in regard to job application procedures, the hiring, advancement, or discharge of employees, employee compensation, job training, and other terms, conditions, and privileges of employment."

The EEOC regulations state that the term "reasonable accommodation" means:

- Modifications to the job application process that enable a qualified disabled individual to be considered for the position.
- Modifications to the work environment or the manner or circumstances under which the position held or desired is customarily performed, that enable a qualified disabled person to perform the essential functions of that position;
- Modifications that enable a disabled employee to enjoy the same benefits and privileges of employment as are enjoyed by non-disabled employees.

The ADA generally adopts the enforcement provisions of Title VII of the Civil Rights Act of 1964, as amended. The EEOC is the designated enforcement arm under both Title VII and the ADA.

Fair Labor Standards Act (FLSA)

There are few federal laws that have as profound an impact on business operations as this act. More than 85% of all non-supervisory employees are now covered by this act, which has been frequently amended by Congress since the first federal minimum wage was established at 25 cents an hour in 1938.

It is commonly said that the FLSA puts a "floor mat under wages" and a "ceiling over hours," but this statement is not precise. The FLSA does establish a minimum wage below which no covered employee may be legally employed. However, it sets a maximum number of hours in any week beyond which a person may be employed only if paid an overtime rate. The FLSA also requires that minimum wage and overtime compensation payments must be made in cash or by check. The sole exception is that costs of board, lodging, and certain other facilities furnished to employees may be deducted from the cash amount paid.

The FLSA requires that applicable minimum wages be paid for all hours worked and that the hours be added in order to ascertain whether overtime pay should be awarded. In general, "hours worked" includes all the time an employee is required to be on duty on the employer's premises or at a prescribed workplace, and all the time the employee is required or permitted to work for the employer.

Note: *Work that is voluntarily performed (such as occurs when an employee remains longer than the prescribed work period to complete an assigned task) is included within the computation of hours worked. Thus, it is the duty of the employer who does not want to pay for this type of "extra" work, to make sure that the employee concludes her work at the end of the assigned work period. The FLSA also includes specific regulations concerning issues such as waiting time, on-call time, preparatory and concluding activities, and attendance at lectures, meetings, training programs, and the like.*

A record must be kept of hours worked each workday and each workweek. A workweek is a regularly reoccurring period of 168 hours in the form of seven consecutive 24-hour periods. Any method of keeping time records is acceptable as long as it is accurate and shows all hours worked. Time clocks are a good means of recording work hours, but they are not required. Rounding to the nearest fraction of an hour (e.g., nearest five minutes or one-tenth or one-fourth) is permitted based upon the rationalization that this agreement averages out over a period of time so that employees are fully paid for all hours they work.

Overtime pay requirements are also provided for in the FLSA. Unless specifically exempted, employees covered by the FLSA must receive overtime pay for hours worked in excess of 40 hours in a workweek at a rate of not less than time and one-half of their regular rate of pay, which may be more but not less than the statutory minimum. (Note: In this instance the state regulations are more restrictive than the FLSA regulations and therefore state rules relative to payment of overtime for eight hours in one workday do prevail.) The regular rate includes all remuneration for employment except reimbursement for expenses incurred on the employer's behalf, premium payments for overtime work, discretionary bonuses, gifts, and payments in the nature of gifts, and payments for occasional periods when no work is performed due to vacation, holiday, or illness.

Certain employees are exempt from minimum wage and overtime pay requirements. The three more notable situations are the so-called "white collar" exemptions (e.g., executive employees, administrative employees, and professional employees). Learners, apprentices, students, and persons subject to child labor regulations are also subject to exemption. Whether an employee is exempt depends on his duties and responsibilities and the salary he is paid. Administrators should note that titles do not make the employee exempt, nor does the fact that he or she is paid a salary rather than on an hourly basis.

Note: *The areas of overtime compensation, recordkeeping, and exemption status are the three most prevalent portions of the FLSA violated by facilities. Administrators must pay attention to the proper payment of overtime, the adequate recordkeeping provisions, and the verification of exempt status of all employees not being paid overtime.*

Child Labor Provisions of the FLSA. Child labor provisions state that the basic minimum age for employment is 16 years. Employment of 14 and 15-year-old youths is permissible but is limited to certain occupations, outside of school hours only, and under specified conditions of work as set forth in the regulations. Administrators are encouraged to pay particular attention to the child labor provisions especially as they relate to the casual employment of school children under the age of 16.

Fair Labor Standards Act Amendments of 1989. On November 29, 1991, the Labor Department's Wage and Hour Division issued a final rule allowing employers to require employees lacking basic skills to spend up to 10 hours in remedial training in addition to their 40-hour workweek without having to pay time and one-half for the overtime. The exemption is limited to those employees who lack a high school diploma or whose reading level or basic skills are at or below the eighth-grade level. Employers must keep records of the time spent in remedial education and amounts paid, which must be at their regular rate of pay. The training must be conducted during a set time and should be away from the employee's regular workstation. The training should be designed to provide reading and basic skills equivalent to the eighth grade level.

Equal Pay Act of 1963. The Equal Pay Act amended the Fair Labor Standards Act to require that men and women performing equal work receive equal compensation. The Equal Pay Act prohibits discrimination on the basis of sex in wage rates between employees performing work in jobs that require equal skill, equal effort, and equal responsibility that are performed under similar working conditions when in the same establishment.

Equal Employment Opportunity Commission (EEOC) and Affirmative Action

Equal employment laws deal with aspects of discrimination and employment because of race, color, religion, national origin, age, sex, pregnancy, or sexual harassment or sexual orientation.

The Equal Employment Opportunity Commission (EEOC) is responsible for enforcing Title VII. It has issued guidelines for the act's interpretation and decides cases brought to it by individuals and groups who believe that they have suffered discrimination.

5

The investigatory responsibility of the EEOC is broad. When it finds reasonable cause that a charge of discrimination is justified, the agency attempts to reach an agreement through persuasion and conciliation. If these efforts fail, the EEOC is empowered to bring a civil action against the employer. The lawsuit does not have to be filed by any particular person or persons but may be on behalf of persons claiming to be aggrieved. Thus, a lawsuit brought by the EEOC could be initiated without specific employee complaints (generally, however, a specific complaint is made). When discrimination is found, courts have ruled that simply providing equal employment opportunity in the future is not enough.

The employer in some instances must "make whole" and "restore the rightful economic status" of all those in the affected class. Courts have the power to order any relief thought to be appropriate, which may include reinstatement or promotion of employees, with or without back pay. Although back pay liability is limited to the two years preceding the filing of the charge with EEOC, some back pay awards, including "class action" suits, have been extraordinarily expensive.

Civil Rights Act of 1964. The cornerstone of equal employment opportunity is a section of this act known as Title VII, which has had an impact on a wide range of employment practices from interviews and hiring procedures to seniority systems and promotion. Title VII prohibits discrimination with respect to compensation and terms, conditions, or privileges of employment because of race, color, religion, sex, national origin, handicap, age, or sexual preference. The thrust of Title VII is twofold: It prohibits discrimination based on factors not related to job qualifications, and it promotes employment based on ability and merit.

In addition, the law seeks to correct past injustices and sources of institutional job bias through mechanisms such as "affirmative action." Title VII of the Civil Rights Act of 1964, as amended and strengthened by legislation in 1972, was the culmination of the struggle of several decades to prohibit racial discrimination by private employers. There was no congressional legislation protecting the civil rights of employees prior to the 1960s; in that decade, Congress enacted several major laws.

The guiding principle behind Title VII is that persons be considered on the basis of individual capacities and not on the basis of any characteristics generally attributed to the group. Also, those individual capacities must be related to the job to be performed, and must not be for the purpose of "screening out" certain individuals. The underlying assumption of Congress is that the factors of race, color, sex, religion, age, sexual preference, disability, or national origin are never criteria in making employment decisions, except in certain limited situations.

While Title VII prohibits a wide variety of discriminatory activities, it does contain several significant exceptions. One major exception is that which permits discrimination based on sex, religion, or national origin in cases where those factors constitute a Bonafide Occupational Qualification (BFOQ). Where such a BFOQ is shown to exist, an employer may consider these factors in employment-related decisions.

Title VII interpretations have significant impacts on employment issues such as interviews, advertising, application forms, employment testing, wage and salary structures, promotion, fringe benefits, and seniority and merit systems.

Civil Rights Act S.1745. On November 21, 1991, President George Bush signed into law and made effective the Civil Rights Act of 1991. Aside from reversing seven U.S. Supreme Court decisions regarding employment discrimination, the law allows

5

for compensatory punitive damages and the right to a jury trial when such damages are sought. Victims of intentional discrimination based on sex, religion, or disability may receive significant damage awards (between $50,000 to $300,000, depending on the size of the workforce). The law also provides for technical assistance and employee training.

Age Discrimination and Employment Act (ADEA). Congress enacted ADEA in 1967. Its purposes are to "promote employment of older persons based on their ability rather than age; to prevent arbitrary age discrimination in employment; to help employers and workers find ways of meeting problems arising from the impact of age on employment." The "older persons" who are protected by the Act are individuals who are at least 40 but younger than 65 years of age. In early 1978, the ADEA was amended to increase the protected upper age to 70 as of January 1, 1979.

The ADEA serves two primary functions: 1) it prohibits arbitrary age discrimination in employment; and 2) it promotes employment based on ability. In this sense, it is similar to Title VII of the 1964 Civil Rights Act.

Under the ADEA, it is unlawful to "fail or refuse to hire or to discharge any individual with respect to his compensation, terms, conditions, or privileges of employment, because of such individual's age." This does not mean that the employer cannot differentiate between employees or prospective applicants when hiring, firing, or promoting. The purpose of ADEA was not to lower performance standards or to make employers ignore differences in qualifications. What the statute requires is that the employer not differentiate solely on the basis of age.

Rehabilitation Act of 1973. The Rehabilitation Act may also legally affect some facilities. Section 504 of the act, merely one long sentence, provides: "No otherwise qualified handicapped individual in the United States … shall, solely by reasons of his handicap, be excluded from the participation in, be denied benefits of, or be subject to discrimination under any program or activity receiving Federal Financial Assistance."

In general, this regulation prohibits employment discrimination against a qualified handicapped employee solely because of handicap. The thrust of the regulation is that employment decisions must be made without regard to physical or mental handicaps that are disqualifying. However, the requirements of the regulation go beyond mere "neutrality" and impose an obligation on the employer to take positive steps to hire and promote qualified handicapped individuals. The regulations define a "qualified handicapped person" as one who "with reasonable accommodation, can perform the essential functions of the job in question." In other words, an employer may not insist that a handicapped employee perform all aspects or functions of a job, but only those that are "essential." The regulations comment that "handicapped persons should not be disqualified simply because they may have difficulty in performing tasks that bear only a marginal relationship to a particular job." Another question raised by the regulations is what kind of "reasonable accommodations" is required? The regulations require such accommodations to the physical or mental impairment of a handicapped applicant or employee unless the accommodation would impose "undue hardship" on the operation of the program. Enforcement of Section 504 is under the U.S. Office of Civil Rights of the Department of Health and Human Services.

Other

In addition to the labor standards, labor relations, and EEO laws, there are also other provisions of both federal and state legislation about which employers must be aware. These include but are not limited to the following:

Veterans Readjustment Assistance Act. This act provides reemployment rights and privileges for veterans to positions that they held prior to their entry into the armed forces. The act requires any employer to rehire a veteran who receives a certificate of satisfactory completion of service if s/he applies for reemployment within 90 days of discharge from training and service or from a hospitalization that continued after his/her discharge for a period up to one year. The U.S. Secretary of Labor aids any person who has satisfactorily completed his/her active duty to seek reemployment and other benefits under this act. The courts specifically have the power to require compliance with the terms of the act and to order compensation to the veteran for any losses of wages or benefits suffered because of the employer's unlawful action.

Immigration Compliance. With the passage of the Immigration Act of 1990, many provisions were added to immigration law. One development is the restructuring of the 1-9 form used by employers to verify the identity and employment eligibility of employees. The law prohibits employers from discriminating against individuals based on national origin or citizenship. In addition, an employer may not require more or different documents to be furnished for verification by any select individual.

Consumer Credit Protection Act. This act places restrictions on the maximum amount of disposable earnings that may be garnished for payments of any debt. Under this act, an employer is prohibited from discharging an employee simply because job earnings have been subjected to one garnishment.

Pregnancy Discrimination Act (PDA). This act prohibits discrimination on the basis of "pregnancy, childbirth and related medical conditions." The law obligates all employers to treat disabilities caused by pregnancy and related conditions the same as other disabilities under any health, disability, insurance, or sick leave plan. A woman cannot be denied a job or promotion merely because she is pregnant or had an abortion. She cannot be fired because of her condition, nor can she be forced to go on leave as long as she is physically capable of working. Women who take maternity leave must be reinstated under the same conditions as employees who return from leaves following other disabilities.

Medicare

The Medicare program was created in 1965 to pay for health services for people age 65 and older. Medicare originated through Title XVIII of the Social Security Act. Though it was initially aimed at the retirement-age population (at the time of its passage age 65 was the mandatory retirement age as well as the age for Social Security eligibility), Medicare was expanded in 1972 to include people of any age with end-stage renal disease (i.e., those receiving dialysis). In 1973 it was expanded to include people of any age who meet Medicare's definition of disability. Ninety percent of Medicare beneficiaries are age 65 and older.

During the ensuing years, Medicare regulations have been modified a number of times in response to changing conditions in the field of health care and for political expediency.

Medicare coverage is divided into two parts. Part A is funded by employer/employee contributions, co-payments, and deductibles. It covers inpatient hospital care, limited skilled nursing facility care, and home health and hospice care for all Medicare beneficiaries. Part B, or supplementary medical insurance (SMI), is funded by premiums, deductibles, and general revenue funds (federal funds). It covers physicians' services and is optional. Members may purchase Part B coverage for a relatively modest monthly premium.

Several health services routinely used by seniors such as routine eye examinations, routine dental care, prescription drugs used on an outpatient basis, and some preventive services are not covered by Medicare. (As of this writing, the debate about instituting prescription drug coverage as a Medicare benefit continues.) Economists estimate that somewhat less than half of a beneficiary's total annual health care expenditures are paid by Medicare. Those who can afford to do so generally purchase supplemental insurance known as Medigap.

Funds used to cover Medicare Part A are placed in a trust fund, the stability of which has been questioned almost since the inception of Medicare! Nonetheless, since this arm of Medicare is funded largely by contributions from those in the workforce, it stands to reason that as the balance of the workforce tilts toward an older age group (such as the "baby boomers," most of whom will have reached retirement age by 2020), the trust fund will be drawn down. The trust fund's viability depends on the size of the contributing workforce and on the longevity of those who use the services provided for by Medicare.

No means test is required for Medicare beneficiaries.

Medicaid

As with Medicare, the Medicaid program was established in 1965 and implemented in 1966. Medicaid is defined as a welfare program that pays for certain mandated health services provided to low-income children and their caretakers. Generally, the caretakers receive or are eligible to receive public assistance funds. Until 1996 these funds were administered through Aid to Families with Dependent Children (AFDC). The Personal Responsibility and Work Opportunity Reconciliation Act of 1996 (PL 104–93) replaced AFDC with the Temporary Assistance for Needy Families (TANF) program. Over time, amendments to the Medicaid act have been made to include people with developmental disabilities and other low-income groups, including the elderly, children, and pregnant women.

Medicaid is funded jointly by the federal and state governments. The state's per capita income determines the amount of federal matching funds. Poorer states have a higher federal match rate than states with higher per capita incomes. States may limit the amount of coverage they provide for each of the basic services mandated under Medicaid.

Unlike Medicare, Medicaid eligibility is means tested. Medicaid pays for a basic set of health services for about 10% of the population. Though children constitute about half (48.8%) of all Medicaid enrollees, they account for approximately 16% of Medicaid expenditures. Blind and disabled persons make up 14.4% of the Medicaid population and account for 37% of the expenditures. More than 14% of Medicare beneficiaries are also enrolled in Medicaid and receive long-term care and other services through Medicaid. Indeed, Medicaid is a major payer for nursing home care.

Medicare and Medicaid are considered legislative "compromises" and are the legacy of Lyndon Johnson's "Great Society." Both came into existence following the government's inability to secure national health insurance, an initiative that had been endorsed as early as 1912 by Teddy Roosevelt during his presidential campaign. Despite efforts over time by leaders of both major political parties—the latest in 1993 with the Health Security Act during the Clinton administration—national health insurance and, by association, universal health care coverage, has yet to be adopted in the United States.

Other Health Care Coverage Programs for Designated Populations

State Children's Health Insurance Program (CHIP). The Balanced Budget Act of 1997 authorized the establishment of CHIP as Title XXI of the Social Security Act. CHIP authorizes the release of federal matching funds for states to initiate and/or expand health insurance assistance for low-income children. CHIP can be linked to Medicaid or can be established as a freestanding program.

Programs for the Medically Indigent. Some states have established programs for the medically indigent. Most are similar to Medicaid in scope; however, they do not receive federal funds.

Programs for Uninsurable Persons. More than half the states have established programs for people with expensive-to-treat chronic conditions whose illnesses prevent them from being covered, because of cost, by traditional insurance programs, even if they would be able to afford the steep premiums.

State Nurse Practice Acts

Each state has in place a nurse practice act that governs the practice of the profession. Practice acts for nursing and other professions are designed first and foremost to safeguard the public. The law is administered by the board of nursing in any given state, province, or territory. Board members represent the professions and the public at large. Laws and regulations under the practice acts specify the conditions under which a nurse may obtain a license to practice nursing in a particular state. Regulations also note the conditions for suspension or revocation of the nurse's license.

States grant reciprocity; that is, a nurse licensed in one state may apply for licensure in another state, pay the requisite fee, and receive a license, provided s/he meets any other criteria specified in the law of a given state, for example, continuing education requirements. Reciprocity is allowed because the state board licensure examination is administered universally; that is, states do not create and administer their own licensing examinations. "Compact" states allow licensure across state lines with no need for a separate application. (See section on "Registration and Licensure" on pg. 117.)

Practice acts also specify the requirements for institutions that provide education for nurses and outline the requisite curriculum. In some states, the state boards are responsible for governance of both registered and practical/vocational nursing practice. In other states, the boards are separate entities.

Institutional Licensure

Institutional licensure is a proposition that would allow an institution to create its own job descriptions and license employees accordingly. There is no merit to the proposal and it has, for all intents and purposes, been laid to rest.

LABOR-MANAGEMENT RELATIONS

Negotiations

Negotiating is the mutual obligation of management and the union to meet at reasonable times and bargain in a good faith effort to reach agreement with respect to conditions of employment affecting employees represented by the union. "Conditions of employment" is a broad term that encompasses personnel policies, practices, and matters affecting working conditions. Certain matters are specifically excluded by law from being considered a condition of employment.

Collective Bargaining

Collective bargaining is defined as an agreement negotiated between a labor union and an employer that sets forth the terms of employment for the employees who are members of the labor union. The agreement may include provisions that pertain to wages, vacation time, working hours, working conditions, and health insurance benefits. The term "collective" acknowledges that the agreements negotiated cover a defined population within an organization and are not "individualized" to each person.

Collective bargaining was once thought anathema to nursing, or to other disciplines that define themselves as professions. However, in 1946, the American Nurses Association (ANA) established its Economic and General Welfare (EG&W) Program with the purpose of improving working conditions for nurses in the United States. The formation of the EG&W Program within the ANA was not without controversy. State nurses associations, as constituents of ANA, replicated EG&W programs at the state level. Some questioned whether an association that speaks for the profession of nursing as a whole could also serve as a union for a segment of its membership. Nonetheless, most collective bargaining agreements covering registered nurses in the United States are negotiated through the labor arm of the ANA-affiliated state nurses associations. California and Massachusetts are notable exceptions and may or may not signal a trend toward total separation of the state organizations that represent nurses. The Massachusetts and California Nurses Associations are no longer affiliates of ANA and are seen primarily as organizations for nurses who work under collective bargaining contracts. In the wake of the schism that caused a break in the traditional organizational structure, two distinct entities now exist in each of these states—the California Nurses Association and the American Nurses Association/California in the Golden State and the Massachusetts Nurses Association and the Massachusetts Association of Registered Nurses in the Bay State.

Grievance and Arbitration
(Source: Chapter XIV: Federal Labor Relations Authority)

The negotiated grievance procedure is a system for resolving disputes. It is a method, established by the union and management, for finding out where problems exist and solving those problems fairly and quickly. Every collective bargaining agreement must contain a negotiated grievance procedure.

A grievance is defined in the collective bargaining agreement and may cover any complaint:

- by any employee concerning any matter relating to the employment of the employee;
- by any labor organization concerning any matter relating to the employment of any employee;
- or by any employee, labor organization, or agency concerning: the effect or interpretation, or a claim of breach, of a collective bargaining agreement; or any claimed violation, misinterpretation, or misapplication of any law, rule, or regulation affecting conditions of employment.

Under negotiated grievance procedures, unions have the right to present and process employee or union grievances. Employees are allowed to present their own grievances (i.e., to represent themselves in the procedure) if they so desire. However, where this happens, the union has the right to be present during the process. Any negotiated grievance not satisfactorily resolved by the grievance process is subject to binding arbitration. Only the union or management may invoke arbitration.

Arbitration is a process in which an impartial third party, the arbitrator, is chosen by the union and management to render a final and binding award after hearing and reviewing the evidence. Because arbitration can be costly, time-consuming, and have unpredictable results, the parties to the dispute should take all necessary steps to attempt to resolve the dispute prior to calling on the arbitrator.

The union or management may file an exception to an arbitrator's award with the Federal Labor Relations Authority. The authority reviews the award to determine whether it is improper because it violates law, rule, or regulation, or on other grounds similar to those applied by federal courts in private sector labor-management relations (e.g., the arbitrator exceeded his or her authority).

The union or management has 30 days beginning on the date of an award to file exceptions with the authority. If no exceptions are filed within that timeframe, then the award becomes final and binding. The refusal of either party to adhere to the award is an unfair labor practice.

National Labor Relations Act

The National Labor Relations Act (NLRA), also known as the Wagner Act, was enacted in 1935 and is the primary law governing relations between unions and employers in the private sector. The law protects workers from the effects of unfair labor practices by employers and requires employers to recognize and bargain collectively with a union that the workers elect to represent them. The NLRA guarantees employees "the right to self-organization, to form, join, or assist labor organizations, to bargain collectively through representatives of their own choosing, and to engage in concerted activities for the purpose of collective bargaining or other mutual aid and protection."

The law was enacted in the wake of widespread strikes and factory takeovers in 1933 and 1934. Violent confrontations occurred between workers trying to form unions and the police and private security forces defending the interests of anti-union employers. Some historians believe that Congress adopted the NLRA primarily in the hopes of averting even greater labor unrest.

By 1945, union membership in the United States reached 35% of the workforce. In response, opponents of organized labor sought to weaken the NLRA. With the passage of the Taft-Hartley Act in 1947, provisions were added to the NLRA that allowed unions to be prosecuted, enjoined, and sued for a variety of activities, including mass picketing and secondary boycotts.

The National Labor Relations Board is an independent federal agency created by Congress to administer the National Labor Relations Act. Through the years, Congress has amended the act and the board and courts have developed a body of law drawn from the statute. The last major revision of the NLRA occurred in 1959, when Congress imposed further restrictions on unions through the Landrum-Griffin Act.

The Landrum-Griffin Act is officially known as the Labor-Management Reporting and Disclosure Act. It resulted from hearings of the Senate committee on improper activities in the fields of labor and management, which uncovered evidence of collusion between dishonest employers and union officials, the use of violence by certain segments of labor leadership, and the diversion and misuse of labor union funds by high-ranking officials. The act grants certain rights to union members and protects their interests by promoting democratic procedures within labor organizations. Union members are protected against abuses by a bill of rights that includes guarantees of freedom of speech and periodic secret elections. Secondary boycotting and organizational and recognition picketing are severely restricted by the act.

Before 1974, it was difficult to discuss labor-management relations laws in the health services field, and especially in the nonprofit sector. All facilities, both proprietary and nonprofit, became subject to the National Labor Relations Act in the late 1950s by virtue of a decision of the National Labor Relations Board. However, in some states, such as California, most nonprofit facilities were not subject to labor organization attempts until after the passage of the Taft-Hartley "hospital exemption." Since the passage of the exemption, all health service institutions are now subject to the Federal Labor Relations Act.

While nonunion facilities may not be concerned on a day-to-day basis with the National Labor Relations Act, facilities with organized unions must carefully attend to the provisions of the NLRA relative to unfair labor practices, boycotts, picketing, and the like.

ACCREDITATION AND CREDENTIALING

Joint Commission on the Accreditation of Healthcare Organizations (JCAHO)

The Joint Commission on the Accreditation of Healthcare Organizations (JCAHO) sets the standards for and accredits over 17,000 health care institutions in the United States. Established in 1951 as the Joint Commission on the Accreditation of Hospitals (JCAHO), JCAHO has grown over the years and expanded its scope to cover far more than acute care hospitals. It now accredits the following types of organizations:

- General, psychiatric, children's and rehabilitation hospitals,
- Health care networks, including Health Maintenance Organizations (HMOs),
- Home care organizations,
- Nursing homes and other long-term care facilities,
- Assisted living facilities,
- Behavioral health care organizations,
- Ambulatory care providers,
- Clinical laboratories.

The corporate members for JCAHO are the American College of Physicians, the American Society of Internal Medicine, the American College of Surgeons, the American Dental Association, the American Hospital Association, and the American Medical Association. The American Nurses Association has not prevailed in its petition for corporate membership. However, nurses are represented on the JCAHO Board of Commissioners. The board is made up of 28 nurses, physicians, consumers, medical directors, administrators, providers, employers, labor representatives, health plan leaders, quality experts, ethicists, health insurance administrators, and educators, representing years of diverse experience in health care, business, and public policy.

There is a relatively long and interesting history of health care organizational review leading up to the formation of JCAHO and explaining the rationale for its

5

corporate membership. Beginning in 1910, Earnest Codman, M.D., proposed that a system was needed to determine whether or not treatments provided in hospitals were effective. Codman suggested that standardization was key to the ability to measure effectiveness. In 1913, the American College of Surgeons (ACS) was established; in 1917, this same body developed and instituted the Minimum Standards for Hospitals, the "parent document" for all subsequent standards. When the first ACS survey was conducted in 1918, 89 of the 692 hospitals reviewed met the requirements of the minimum standards. Over the years, the other medical and hospital associations that now form the JCAHO corporate membership were incorporated into the structure of the organization.

JCAHO strengthened its survey approach over the years and, in 1965, with the passage of the Social Security amendment that established Medicare, those hospitals that held JCAHO accreditation were "deemed" in compliance with most of the Medicare Conditions of Participation for Hospitals. Thus, even though it is a private organization and charges for its services, JCAHO, by virtue of its reputation and the oversight work it does relative to quality and effectiveness, has become a surrogate for public sector (government) accreditation. Its name change in 1987 reflects JCAHO's expanded scope of activities.

JCAHO is now at another crossroad in its journey. In 1993, it shifted focus from standards that measure an organization's capability to perform to those that determine its actual performance. In 1996, JCAHO and the Occupational Safety and Health Administration (OSHA) joined in a three-year partnership to help health care organizations meet accreditation expectations that promote health and safety for health care workers. In 1998, JCAHO, the American Medical Accreditation Program, and the National Committee for Quality Assurance (NCQA) announced a collaborative effort designed to coordinate performance measurement activities across the entire health care system. The agreement establishes the Performance Measurement Coordinating Council to ensure that measurement-driven assessment processes are efficient, consistent, and useful. In 1999, JCAHO revised its mission statement to focus on patient safety: "The mission of the Joint Commission is to continuously improve the safety and quality of care provided to the public through the provision of health care accreditation and related services that support performance improvement in health care organizations."

JCAHO and the institutions that seek accreditation through it have been criticized over the years for the intensity of pre-survey preparation. The alleged promise to the public is that accredited institutions will be in a constant state of readiness with regard to quality of care and patient safety. How this status can be shown was codified in 2000 with the revision of JCAHO's Random Unannounced Survey Policy. No advance notice for random unannounced surveys is provided to the organization; unannounced surveys may be conducted from nine to 30 months following the triennial full survey. The scope and focus of the unannounced survey will vary based on information relating to recommendations made during the organization's previous triennial survey, known sentinel events, and known performance.

Further revision of JCAHO's approach is underway. By 2004, JCAHO will have implemented its "Shared Visions—New Pathways" initiative, which will highlight care systems critical to the safety and quality of patient care. The "new pathways" include:

5

- Mid-cycle self-assessment during which the health care organization will evaluate its own compliance with the applicable standards and develop a plan of correction for identified areas of noncompliance.
- Pre-survey review of organization-specific information, such as ORYX core measure data, sentinel event information, and MedPar data, through an automated process to identify critical processes relevant to patient safety and health care quality.
- Substantial consolidation of the standards to reduce the paperwork and documentation burden of the survey process and increase its focus on patient safety and health care quality.
- On-site evaluation of standards compliance in relation to the care experience of actual patients.
- Revision of individual organization performance reports to provide performance information not included in the current reports.
- Active engagement of physicians in the new accreditation process

Current JCAHO Standards are divided into three categories and 15 sections, each with several subsections.

Joint Commission on the Accreditation of Healthcare Organizations

Category	Section
1. Patient-Focused Functions	1. Patients Rights and Organizational Ethics (RI) 2. Patient Education (PE) 3. Care of Patients (TX) 4. Patient Education (PF) 5. Continuum of Care (CC)
2. Organization-Focused Functions	6. Improving Organizational Performance (PI) 7. Leadership (LD) 8. Management of the Environment of Care (EC) 9. Management of Human Resources (HR) 10. Management of Information (IM) 11. Surveillance, Prevention, and Control of Infection (IC)
3. Structures with Functions	12. Governance (GO) 13. Management (MA) 14. Medical Staff (MS) 15. Nursing (NR)

As with most large public organizations, JCAHO has a presence on the World Wide Web. JCAHO's robust Web site provides a wealth of information for health care professionals and the public alike.

5

Specialty Accreditation (e.g., Home Health, Long-Term Care, Rehabilitation, Substance Abuse)

Though JCAHO is the best known of the accrediting bodies, other organizations also offer accreditation for various specialty care institutions or services.

CCAC/CARF

In January 2003, the Continuing Care Accreditation Commission (CCAC) merged with the Commission on Accreditation of Rehabilitation Facilities (CARF); both are nonprofit organizations. CCAC is the only accrediting body in the United States for aging services continuums, including continuing care retirement communities. CARF accredits adult day services, assisted living, behavioral health, employment and community services, and medical rehabilitation services. Both organizations promote the adoption of rigorous standards for the care of the special populations that are the focus of their accreditation activities.

NCQA

The National Committee for Quality Assurance (NCQA) is the accrediting body for managed care organizations. It surveys the following types of facilities: managed behavioral health care organizations, managed care organizations, preferred provider organizations, and so forth. Similar to JCAHO, NCQA publishes "report cards" indicating the comparative quality of various organizations measured against established standards (**www.ncqa.org**).

NCQA sponsors, supports, and maintains the Health Plan Employer Data Information Set (HEDIS). HEDIS is a set of standardized performance measures designed to ensure that purchasers and consumers have the information they need to reliably compare the performance of managed health care plans. The performance measures in HEDIS are related to significant public health issues such as cancer, heart disease, smoking, asthma, and diabetes. HEDIS also includes a standardized survey of consumers' experiences that evaluates plan performance in areas such as customer service, access to care, and claims possessing.

SAMHSA

The Substance Abuse and Mental Health Services Administration (SAMHSA) was established in October 1992. Its intent is to strengthen the nation's health care capacity to provide prevention, diagnosis, and treatment services for substance abuse and mental illnesses. SAMHSA works in partnership with states, communities, and private organizations to address the needs of people with substance abuse and mental illnesses as well as the community risk factors that contribute to these illnesses. It does not directly accredit programs or facilities.

SAMHSA serves as the umbrella organization for the Center for Mental Health Services (CMHS), the Center for Substance Abuse Prevention (CSAP), and the Center for Substance Abuse Treatment (CSAT).

5

AAAHC

The Accreditation Association for Ambulatory Care (AAAHC) is an organization whose energies are directed to improving practice in ambulatory care facilities. In January 2003, AAAHC and the Joint Commission on Accreditation of Healthcare Organizations (JCAHO) signed a cooperative accreditation agreement, allowing AAAHC accreditation to fulfill JCAHO standards for ambulatory care organizations in certain situations.

Credentialing

Registration and Licensure

The responsibilities of state boards of nursing include a duty to protect the public. The boards control the licensure process and as such "register" nurses to practice under the conditions set forth in regulations. Because nurses occupy a position of trust in society, the state boards also have a duty to protect the public from unscrupulous or unlawful practice by licensed nurses. Sanctions exist and licenses can be revoked or suspended for those who violate the law or who are convicted of certain crimes.

Licensure is "the process by which an agency of state government grants permission to an individual to engage in a given profession upon finding that the applicant has attained the essential degree of competency necessary to perform a unique scope of practice" (National Council of State Boards of Nursing, 2001).

Prior to sitting for the licensure examination, the candidate must demonstrate that s/he meets the qualifications required to practice nursing within a defined scope (RN, LVN/LPN). Only those who meet the criteria of licensure are permitted to use the title for their role. Provision for disciplinary action in the event of violation of the law assures protection of the public.

Nurses are licensed to practice in a given state and state boards of nursing govern licensure. While each state retains its sovereignty over the licensing process for its jurisdiction, all states now grant reciprocity to nurses who move from one state to another if the nurse (RN or LPN/LVN) applies for and is granted a license to practice in the second state. This was not always the case. In decades past, depending on the regulations of a particular state, a graduate nurse may have taken a state board examination in one state, only to have to complete the process in another state when s/he changed residence.

"Nurse compact" legislation is a growing trend. Compact legislation allows the nurse who is licensed in one "compact" state to practice in other "compact" states without the need to apply for licensure in the second (or third or fourth) state. Model legislative language exists and in time, it is expected that most states will endorse the compact approach to licensure recognition, though holdouts will likely remain for political or economic reasons.

Given the mobility of society in general, the proliferation of "traveling nurse" services, and the advent of nurse tele-advice centers that process calls from clients from throughout the country, the compact approach seems reasonable. On the other hand, the compact means that state agencies must give up some measure of autonomy and parochial control of practice within their jurisdictions.

The National Council of State Boards of Nursing (NCSBN) oversees the development of the NCLEX-RN® and NCLEX-PN® examinations. The "state board" examinations, once completed with paper and pencil, are now taken using a computer. Pass scores are set and, once achieved during the testing process, the test is stopped. The test measures cognitive ability and requires that the applicant demonstrate the ability to process complex situations. The examination is defined as a "power" test as opposed to a "speed" test. That is, though the test must be completed within the allotted five-hour timeframe, speed of response to discreet questions within the test is not a factor in scoring the test. The test is designed from the perspective of "client needs" and is divided into four main sections and 10 subsections. The four main sections are: 1) safe, effective care environment; 2) health promotion and maintenance; 3) psychosocial integrity; and 4) physiological integrity.

Currently, graduates of diploma, baccalaureate, and associate degree programs in nursing sit for the same examination. The pass rate for graduates of each type of program appears to be remarkably similar over time.

Certification

Certification provides recognition of nurses who meet specified requirements, usually for a particular field or clinical specialty, but does not include a legal scope of practice. Certification is generally voluntary; however, many state boards use professional certification as a requirement for granting authority for advance practice registered nurses (e.g., nurse practitioners). As certification is increasingly recognized as a hallmark of specialty practice, more organizations are at the very least stating "certification in specialty preferred" as part of the employment process.

Other Issues

Advanced Practice

In 2000, the Delegate Assembly of the National Council of State Boards of Nursing (NCSBN) passed the Uniform Advanced Practice Registered Nurse Licensure/Authority to Practice Requirements. The requirements include: 1) unencumbered RN license; 2) graduation from a graduate-level advanced practice program accredited by a national accrediting body; 3) current certification by a national certifying body in the advanced practice specialty appropriate to educational preparation; and 4) maintenance of certification or evidence of maintenance of competence.

The NCSBN 2002 Position Paper on the Regulation of Advance Practice Nursing offers guidance for state regulatory bodies. The intent is to assure consistency in education, licensure, certification requirements, and practice scope throughout the country. Realization of the goals set forth in the position paper will foster public safety and permit greater mobility for advance practice nurses. The full text of the position paper is available on the NCSBN website at www.ncsbn.org/.

PROFESSIONAL AND INSTITUTIONAL LIABILITY

Insurance

Two types of liability are of concern to those in the health professions: personal liability and corporate liability. **Personal liability** holds that individuals are responsible for their own actions. **Vicarious** liability is an extension of personal liability and holds that certain parties may not be negligent themselves but their negligence is assumed because of association with the negligent individual. **Corporate liability** holds that an organization is responsible for its conduct.

Corporate liability encompasses: 1) the duty to hire and maintain an adequate number of qualified, competent staff members; 2) the duty to provide safe, adequate equipment; 3) the duty to maintain safety in the physical environment.

Health care organizations are, by the nature of their business, heavily insured to protect against liability, and, by extension, their employees are also insured. The doctrine of *respondeat superior* (let the master speak) allows the courts to hold employers responsible for the actions of the organization's employees when the employees are performing services for the organization. This concept sometimes gives nurses and other health care professionals a false sense of security in that they assume they cannot be sued individually in the case of actual or perceived wrongdoing. This is false reasoning. Patients may sue both the institution and the individual practitioner. Thus, nurses are advised to carry their own personal liability insurance.

Documentation

The need for precise, accurate documentation has been reinforced repeatedly in the field of nursing. "If it's not documented, it's not done," is an oft-repeated mantra within the profession. New challenges lie ahead as computerized documentation systems become more widespread without benefit of standardized rules, processes, and technical languages. Though such guidelines will come in time through various regulatory bodies, the initial products are being activated at the institutional level. At the present time, electronic documentation systems are no more consistent than their paper and pen counterparts!

5

Malpractice and Negligence

The terms negligence and malpractice are sometimes confused with one another or assumed to be synonymous. This is not the case. Negligence is the failure to do what a reasonably careful and prudent person would do under the same or like circumstances (omission), or the doing of something that a reasonably careful and prudent person would not do under the same or like circumstances (commission). Briefly, negligence is the failure to exercise reasonable or ordinary care.

Malpractice goes beyond negligence. Four elements must be present for malpractice to occur:

- duty (How would a reasonable and prudent provider behave under the same circumstances?);
- breach of duty (Did the provider breach the standard of care in this particular situation?);
- causation (Was the unreasonable, careless or inappropriate behavior on the part of the provider the proximate cause of the injury or insult?); and
- injury (Did injury to the patient/client occur?). If any one of these elements cannot be proved "beyond a reasonable doubt," then a malpractice claim may be dismissed.

Risk Management

Risk management has taken on new importance in the field of health care, particularly with mandates and commitments related to disclosure of adverse events. Risk management is an organization-wide service that identifies and takes corrective action to reduce jeopardy to the establishment, patients, and staff. It is a problem-focused approach with a clear intent to reduce the frequency and severity of accidents and injuries.

Key elements of a risk management program include:

- Identification of potential hazards and inspection to locate problem areas.
- Review of monitoring systems to assure their integrity. Monitoring systems include incident reports, questionnaires, minutes of committees, oral complaints, and audits.
- Analysis and categorization of incidents that result in actual or potential adverse outcomes.
- Review and tracking of laws related to patient safety, legal codes, and care.
- Elimination of risk wherever possible.
- Identification of education and training needs relative to risk management.
- Preparing administrative reports to keep the executives of the organization appraised of risk management findings and preventive and corrective actions.

The monumental significance of risk management was highlighted with the 1999 release of the Institute of Medicine (IOM) report entitled "To Err Is Human:

Building a Safer Health Care System." The report focused on the need to improve safety systems within health care.

The IOM highlighted the risks of medical care in the United States and shocked both the professional and public sectors with its estimates of the magnitude of medical errors resulting in death (44,000 to 98,000 deaths per year) and other serious events.

Three months after publication of the IOM report, an interagency federal government group, the Quality Interagency Coordination Task Force (QuIC), released its response, "Doing What Counts for Patient Safety: Federal Actions to Reduce Medical Errors and Their Impact." The report prompted legislative and regulatory initiatives designed to document errors and begin the search for solutions. The report listed more than a hundred action items to be undertaken by federal agencies.

The Agency for Healthcare Research and Quality (AHRQ), the federal agency devoted to research that promotes patient safety, was charged with continuing "the development and dissemination of evidence-based, best safety practices to provider organizations."

Those working on the project began by defining "patient safety practices" as "a type of process or structure whose application reduces the probability of adverse events resulting from exposure to the health care system across a range of diseases and procedures." This definition is consistent with a philosophical framework for patient safety, which holds that systemic change will be far more productive in reducing medical errors than will targeting and punishing individual providers. The approach used by the researchers in this process is known as "evidence-based" review.

The review focuses on hospital care as a starting point because the risks associated with hospitalization are significant, the strategies for improvement are better documented there than in other health care settings, and the importance of patient trust is paramount. The AHRQ report also considers evidence regarding other sites of care, such as nursing homes, ambulatory care, and patient self-management.

The results of the study will be used by the National Quality Forum (NQF) to identify a set of proven patient safety practices that should be used by hospitals. NFQ's identification of these practices allows patients to evaluate the actions their hospitals and/or health care facilities have taken to improve safety.

Employee Impairment

Statistics indicate that the incidence of impairment within the ranks of health care employees and practitioners mirrors that of the occurrence of impairment in the general public. The figure is set at 10%.

Most state licensing boards and medical societies have special programs for treating impaired practitioners. Program staffs work with impaired practitioners throughout the course of active treatment and recovery. The intent is to maintain the practitioner in her/his profession whenever possible. In the past, a veil of secrecy surrounded the interventions aimed at helping impaired practitioners. With the increased need to be accountable to the public, this veil has been lifted with the identification of practitioners made public under certain circumstances. For example, the names of nurses whose licenses have been suspended or revoked for cause are a matter of public record; disclosure is under the auspices of state boards of nursing.

There is now a link between the Americans with Disability Act (ADA) and impaired employees who have completed a drug/alcohol rehabilitation program. The ADA protects the person who has been successfully rehabilitated and is no longer using drugs/alcohol or the employee who is participating in a supervised rehabilitation program.

Fraud, Abuse and Waste—Corporate Compliance

Corporate compliance initiatives have become a mainstay of the health care business environment. While the amount of "legitimate" waste in the health care industry is the focus of those involved with the economics and quality of health care, fraud and abuse are in another dimension altogether. Health care organizations are required to have in place corporate compliance systems that are designed to prevent legal and regulatory violations, to identify fraud and abuse within the health care system, and to establish principles that demonstrate an organization's commitment to the highest standards of excellence in its business practices.

For the purposes of the health care system, **fraud** means an intentional deception or misrepresentation made by a person with the knowledge that the deception could result in some unauthorized benefit to himself or some other person. It includes any act that constitutes fraud under applicable federal or state law.

Abuse means provider practices that are inconsistent with sound fiscal, business, or medical practices, and result in an unnecessary cost or in reimbursement for services that are not medically necessary or fail to meet professionally recognized standards for health care.

Health Insurance Portability and Accountability Act

HIPAA is the acronym for the Health Insurance Portability and Accountability Act of 1996, known also as the Kennedy-Kassenbaum Bill (Public Law 104–191). The law was passed in August 1996, and portions of it having to do with the electronic exchange and protection of health care data have generated controversy ever since.

Title I of the law allows persons to qualify immediately for comparable health insurance coverage when they change their employment relationships. There is little disagreement with the "goodness" of this element of the law.

Title II of the law gives the Department of Health and Human Services (HHS) the authority to mandate the use of standards for the electronic exchange of health care data; to specify what medical and administrative code sets should be used within those standards; to require the use of national identification systems for health care patients, providers, payers (or plans), and employers (or sponsors); and to specify the types of measures required to protect the security and privacy of personally identifiable health care information. As of April 2003, health care systems are required to show evidence of compliance with the intent of the law as it pertains to the exchange of data and the notification of such exchange.

There is no simple explanation for the intricacies of HIPAA. It is safe to say that health care administrators will be involved with the implementation and interpretation of its privacy rules for years to come. Whether or not the safeguards of personal health status information promised to the public through the enactment of HIPAA will be realized as intended is yet to be determined.

POLITICS

Political Process

Politics is generally thought of in terms of campaigns, philosophies, control of government, achievement of elected office, and so forth. However, broadly defined, politics is the ability to influence events in order to achieve an intended objective. Nurses have yet to fully realize their collective political power, whether in the community arena or within the work or academic settings. Nonetheless, things are changing and nurses are gaining sophistication in the use of the political process.

Nurses have much to contribute to the development of health policy and will do so more readily as they develop political expertise. Their intimate and expert knowledge of the intricacies of the health care setting serves them well. When combined with a deeper comprehension of the systems and business issues facing health care and the intent to build coalitions within and outside of the nursing profession, they will gain greater power and political clout.

Power

Power is the capacity to act and the energy to mobilize resources in order to create change. Whether power has a positive or a negative connotation depends on how it is used. Several types of power available to leaders have been identified.

- **Legitimate** power suggests that the leader has the right or authority to tell others what to do. The reciprocal nature of legitimate power obligates employees to comply with legitimate orders.
- **Reward** power is exercised over others when the leader has the ability to compensate others in some way. Compensation need not be monetary.
- **Coercive** power indicates that the leader who exercises this type of power has the ability to punish those who are noncompliant.
- **Referent** power means that the leader has characteristics that appeal to others. People comply because they admire the leader or have a desire for approval.

5

■ **Expert** power means that the leader has certain expertise or knowledge. People comply because they believe in or can otherwise gain from affiliation with the person with expert power.

All sources of power are potentially important and the assumption is that the most powerful leaders are those who have high legitimate, reward, or coercive power. However, one should not underestimate the strength of referent and expertise power. These sources of power are more closely related to personal motivation and may, in the long run, make a greater and more lasting difference within a company or organization. Nor is it necessarily the leaders whose names are well known or who sit atop the organizational chart who exert the most power of this type.

Lobbying

Through formal lobbying activities, nurses attempt to influence legislative bodies or individuals at the federal, state, district, or local level to support legislation seen as beneficial to the profession as a whole, to particular interest groups, or to the public at large. Various factions within nursing may, at times, find themselves on opposite ends of the spectrum relative to the positions they take on a particular bill or act. Through political action committees (PACs), nurses are able to contribute financially to help assure that their position is heard.

Nursing organizations may employee paid lobbyists to advance their agenda in Washington or at the state house. Lobbyists are not necessarily nurses, but they do understand and work toward achieving the outcome specified by the nursing organization that employs them.

The public persona of the lobbyist may differ from that displayed by the lobbyist behind the scenes where the art of negotiation and compromise may be practices to gain the "best" position in a given circumstance.

Nurses and others who work on their behalf employ the same techniques used by the professional lobbyist in their daily encounters. This is particularly true of those in managerial or executive roles who find the political process both rewarding and essential to achieving organizational, professional, and personal goals.

Networking

Networking is the exchange of information or services among individuals, groups, or institutions. Nurses gain significant benefit from networking activities that take place within or between organizations or as part of professional activities. Various associations offer the nurse manager or nurse executive rich opportunities to network with colleagues. Nurses build their collective power through the creation of formal and informal networks.

"Diffusion of innovation," a construct explored by Everett Rogers and detailed earlier in this study guide, takes place largely through networking.

CONTRACTS AND AGREEMENTS

A contract, broadly defined, is an agreement between two or more parties. Contracts may be formal, that is, written and executed, or informal, such as a "handshake" or a verbal agreement.

Types

Service

Service contracts are negotiated to assure that equipment is cared for as it should be and that those who agree to provide a service honor their commitment to do so. The service is generally intangible in that the exchange occasioned by the contract has no physical dimension.

In another sense, a contract to provide health care service exists between patients and providers or between members and health plans.

Educational

Educational contracts define the expectations that learners and instructors have of one another, or the exchange of services that educational institutions and health care institutions will provide for one another, or the outcome that a learner intends to achieve upon engaging in a learning activity.

Labor

Labor contracts contain the provisions agreed to by both parties to the contract—the labor union and the management of an organization. Labor contracts typically include the following elements: security clause, a management's rights clause, seniority provisions, wages and hours, fringe benefits, layoff or reduction in force language, insurance, retirement, professional issues, dues structure, and so forth. Contracts are not acted on until members of the affected union ratify them through the voting process. Ratification occurs when a simple majority agrees to accept the conditions of the contract.

Administration of Contracts and Agreements

Administration of union contracts is the responsibility of the designated union representative. The representative is charged with providing fair and equal representation for all members of the unit. The representative explains the provisions of the contract to the members of the union. The union representative also participates in the grievance process as this becomes necessary.

5

Online Resources

The following websites are among the many that offer a wealth of information to nurses in leadership positions.

- Agency for Health Care Research and Quality
  www.ahrq.gov (accessed 12/07/06)

- Alliance of Community Health Plans
  www.achp.org/default.asp (accessed 12/07/06)

- American Association of Colleges of Nursing — End-of Life Nursing Education Consortium
  www.aacn.nche.edu/ELNEC/ (accessed 12/07/06)
- American Nurses Association Web Portal
  www.nursingworld.org/ (accessed 12/07/06)

- ANCC Magnet Recognition
  www.nursecredentialing.org/magnet/index.html (accessed 12/07/06)

- American Society for Quality
  www.asq.org/index.html (accessed 12/07/06)

- Baldridge National Quality Program (BNQP)
  www.quality.nist.gov/ (accessed 12/07/06)

- Health Insurance Portability and Accountability Act (HIPAA) Privacy Rules
  http://privacyruleandresearch.nih.gov/pr_02.asp (accessed 12/07/06)

- Health Resources and Services Administration
  www.hrsa.gov (accessed 12/07/06)

- Internet Healthcare Coalition (Code of Ethics)
  www.ihealthcoalition.org/ethics/ehcode.html (accessed 12/07/06)

- Joint Commission on Accreditation of Healthcare Organization
  www.jcaho.org/ (accessed 12/07/06)

- National Council of States Boards of Nursing, Inc
  www.ncsbn.org/public/index.htm (accessed 12/07/06)

- National Database of Nursing Quality Indicators
  www.nursingquality.org/ (accessed 12/07/06)

- National Labor Relations Board
  www.nlrb.gov (accessed 12/07/06)

- National Quality Forum
  www.qualityforum.org (accessed 12/07/06)

- OD Network Online
  www.odnetwork.org (accessed 12/07/06)

- US Department of Labor Occupational Safety and Health Administration
  www.osha.gov (accessed 12/07/06)

- United States Government Web Portal
  www.firstgov.gov (accessed 12/07/06)

- University of Washington School of Medicine/Ethics in Medicine
  http://depts.washington.edu/bioethx/ (accessed 12/07/06)

A

APPENDIX B

References

American Nurses Association. (2003). *Scope and standards for nursing administration*. Washington, DC: American Nurses Publishing.

American Nurses Association. (2000). *Scope and standards of practice for nursing professional development*. Washington, DC: American Nurses Publishing.

Barton, P. (2003). *Understanding the U.S. health services system* (2nd ed.). Chicago: Health Administration Press.

Bateman, T., & Snell, S. (2002). *Management: Competing in the new era* (5th ed). Boston: McGraw-Hill Irwin.

Benner, P. (1984). From novice to expert: Excellence and power in clinical nursing practice. Menlo Park, CA: Addison-Wesley.

Benner, P., Tanner, C., & Chesla, C. (1996). *Expertise in nursing practice: Caring, clinical judgment and ethics*. New York: Springer.

Bizony, N. (1999). Interest-based negotiation: Moving beyond our scarcity model. OD Practitioner Online. Retrieved May 17, 2003, from http://www.odnetwork.org/odponline/vol31n3/interestbased.html.

Burns, N., & Grove, S. (2002). *Understanding nursing research* (3rd ed.). Philadelphia: W. B. Saunders

Connor, D. (1995). *Managing at the speed of change: How resilient managers succeed and prosper where others fail*. New York: Villard Books.

Deming, W. E. (2000). *Out of the crisis*. Boston: MIT Press.

Dye, C. (2000). *Leadership in healthcare: Values at the top*. Chicago: Health Administration Press.

Fisher, R., Ury, W., & Patton, B. (Eds.). (1991). Getting to yes: Negotiating agreement without giving in. New York: Penguin.

Glaser, J. (1997). *Three realms of managed care: Societal, institutional, individual — Resources for group reflection and action*. Lanham, MD: Sheed & Ward.

Greenwald, H., & Beery, W. (2002). *Health for all: Making community collaboration work*. Chicago: Health Administration Press.

Griffith, J., & White, K. (2002). *The well-managed healthcare organization* (5th ed.). Chicago: Health Administration Press.

Harris, M. (1998). *Basic statistics for behavioral science research* (2nd ed.). Boston: Allyn & Bacon.

Irving, A., & Hiss, S. (2001, March). Impaired healthcare practitioners: Some legal and risk management considerations. *Risk Management Briefings*.

Kolcaba, K. (2002). *Comfort theory and practice: A vision for holistic health care and research*. New York: Springer Publishing Co.

Longest, B. (2002). *Health policymaking in the United States* (3rd ed.). Chicago: Health Administration Press.

Longest, B., Rakich, J., & Darr, K. (2000). *Managing health services organizations and systems* (4th ed.). Baltimore: Health Professions Press.

Marquis, B., & Huston, C. (2002). *Leadership roles and management functions in nursing: Theory and application.* Philadelphia: Lippincott, Williams & Wilkins.

Marriner-Tomey, A., & Alligood, M. (2002). *Nursing theorists and their work* (5th ed.). St. Louis: Mosby.

Morrison, I. (2002). *Health care in the new millennium: Vision, values, and leadership* (1st ed.). San Francisco: Jossey-Bass.

Munhall, P. (2001). *Nursing research: A qualitative perspective* (3rd ed.). Boston: Jones & Bartlett.

Phillips, J. (1992). *How to think about statistics* (Rev. ed.). New York: Freeman.

Potter, P., & Perry, A. (2001). *Fundamentals of nursing* (5th ed.). St. Louis: Mosby.

Price, Waterhouse, Coopers. (2002, April). *The factors fueling rising healthcare costs.* [Study prepared for the American Association of Health Plans].

Puskin, D. (2001, September 30). Telemedicine: Follow the money. *Online Journal of Issues in Nursing.* Retrieved December 6, 2006, from http://www.nursingworld.org/ojin/topic16/tpc16_1.htm.

Schermerhorn, J., Hunt, J., & Osborn, R. (1995). *Scope and standards for nursing administration.* Washington, DC: American Nurses Publishing.

Shi, E., & Singh, D. (2001). *Delivering health care in America: A systems approach* (2nd ed.) Boston: Jones & Bartlett.

Spath, P. (Ed.). (2002). *Guide to effective staff development in health care organizations: A systems approach to successful training.* San Francisco: Jossey-Bass.

Sullivan, E., & Decker, P. (2000). Effective leadership and management in nursing (5th ed.). Upper Saddle River, NJ: Prentice Hall.

Swansburg, R., & Swansburg, R. J. (2002). *Introduction to management and leadership for nurse managers* (3rd ed.). Boston: Jones & Bartlett.

Tappen, R. (2001). *Essentials of nursing leadership and management.* Philadelphia: F. A. Davis Co.

Walton, M., & Deming, E. (1988). *Deming management method.* New York: Perigee.

Withrow, S. (2001). *Managing HIPAA compliance: Standards for electronic transmission.* Chicago: Health Administration Press.

Woodworth, G. (2003, Winter). Technology and standards — 2003: The year of medical paperwork simplification. Retrieved December 6, 2006 from http://www.himss.org/asp/ContentRedirector.asp?ContentID=25655.

B

Practice Test

1. In management by objectives:
   a. managers determine the goals employees should accomplish.
   b. employees independently set the goals they should achieve.
   c. managers are supportive, using counseling and coaching.
   d. managers encourage employees to set high goals and assume responsibility for their achievement.

2. In assessing the philosophy for nursing services for possible revision, the nurse executive is most heavily influenced by the organization's:
   a. mission statement.
   b. consumer surveys.
   c. financial resources.
   d. policy statements.

3. In planning strategies to prevent stagnation and promote renewal in the nursing division, which action would most likely result in the desired outcome?
   a. Developing a program for recruitment of young talent.
   b. Rewarding employees by promoting from within.
   c. Having set pay increases mandated annually.
   d. Using longevity to determine committee selection.

4. In planning for change, the successful change agent makes a commitment to:
   a. help followers arrive at total consensus regarding the change.
   b. encourage subgroup opposition to change so many viewpoints can be heard.
   c. utilize change by drift if resistance to change is too strong.
   d. be available to support those affected by change until refreezing occurs.

5. In planning marketing strategies for the new oncology wing, the nurse executive remembers that the best approach is to:
   a. develop surveys of patient's likes and dislikes.
   b. advertise the unit through print and television media.
   c. provide quality patient care and family support.
   d. hire an all-licensed nursing staff.

6. Needs assessment and analysis of the organization's strengths and weaknesses help to determine:
   a. an organization's market share.
   b. the risks of over-marketing.
   c. the implementation of a market plan.
   d. the needs of the clients who are likely to use the services of the organization.

7. Decentralized organizational structure promotes decision making that:
   a. allows problems to be solved at the level they occur.
   b. encourages decisions to be made by top-level hierarchy.
   c. limits communication to managers at various levels.
   d. assigns responsibility at the highest practical level.

8. When planning for managed care, which goals are most appropriate for the nurse manager?
   a. Clinical outcomes should occur within a prescribed timeframe.
   b. Case managers should not function as providers of patient care.
   c. Managed care practice should be unit based and unit specific.
   d. Outcome management should be carried out for each patient.

9. During a strategic planning committee meeting to develop futuristic goals for technology, several unit managers spend a considerable amount of time discussing current staffing problems. As chairperson of this committee, the nurse executive's primary action is to:
   a. take the remainder of the meeting time to discuss the staffing with all members.
   b. adjourn the meeting and reschedule at a time when there are less staffing problems.
   c. request that committee members return to discussing the items on the agenda.
   d. excuse those discussing staffing from the committee meeting.

10. Critical pathways outline a patient's expected progress from admission to discharge and are part of
    a. functional nursing.
    b. primary care nursing.
    c. case management
    d. team nursing.

11. An effective patient classification system:
    a. eliminates most staffing problems.
    b. decreases the amount of overtime.
    c. matches staff resources to patient care needs.
    d. eliminates the need for adjustment or review.

12. When using a patient classification system, the nurse executive should understand that such systems:
    a. are used to solve unit staffing shortages.
    b. use nonvariable nursing care hours.
    c. are designed to eliminate human error.
    d. are periodically reevaluated.

13. In evaluating the Nursing Department's Total Quality Management (TOM) program, the administrator understands that the underlying principle of TOM:
    a. has the customer as the focal element upon which production and service depend.
    b. assumes that inspection of and removal of errors leads to quality.
    c. is based on the premise that the organization knows what is best for the consumer.
    d. has a guiding purpose of organizational efficacy and cost containment.

14. When evaluating the nursing service philosophy, the most important thing to ascertain is that the philosophy:
    a. is congruent with the mission of the organization.
    b. can be implemented in a cost-effective manner.
    c. flows from organizational goals.
    d. is brief and simply worded.

15. In determining quality control for marketing, the most qualitative measurement would be:
    a. general satisfaction levels of patients.
    b. morbidity and mortality statistics.
    c. nursing care hours per patient day.
    d. average length of stay.

16. To adhere to the principles of responsible accounting, the nursing executive ensures that:
    a. nursing service is accountable for nursing-generated revenues, expenses, and liabilities.
    b. each nursing service manager is responsible for turning in his or her budget on time.
    c. each department head meets with the financial officer prior to submitting a budget
    d. all nursing service accounting is honest, reviewed in a timely fashion, and accurate.

17. This year's operating budget for 3 South is $1.4 million. Eighty percent of the budget is allocated for personnel costs (wages, taxes, and benefits). What is the dollar amount of this year's personnel budget for 3 South?
    a. $980 thousand
    b. $1.12 million
    c. $1.18 million
    d. $1.24 million

C

18. Next year the total budget allocation for 3 South will increase to $1.6 million. However, the personnel costs will also increase by 5% compared with the current year. Based on this assumption, personnel costs next year will be:
    a. $ 1.28 million
    b. $ 1.36 million
    c. $ 1.42 million
    d. $ 1.48 million

19. In the above scenario, as the final round in the budgeting process for next year takes place, the manager is asked to cut the non-payroll budget by 10%. This means that the non-payroll operating budget figure for the coming year is now:
    a. $ 216,000
    b. $ 224,000
    c. $ 230,000
    d. $ 240,000

20. The nurse executive who is implementing a hospital's cost containment program should realize that the most important step is to:
    a. develop an inservice curriculum that focuses on cost containment.
    b. develop methods for determining nursing care costs for each patient category.
    c. negotiate redistribution of non-nursing tasks to other departments.
    d. ask nurses to become a part of the decision-making process in the areas of patient care, unit management, and hospital governance.

21. Important considerations in the fiscal management of nursing care delivery systems include:
    a. workload and nursing hours per patient per day.
    b. patient care requirements and physician recommendations.
    c. nursing and non-nursing salaries.
    d. job satisfaction and productivity.

22. Costs per unit of service will increase as:
    a. volume decreases below the break-even point.
    b. volume increases
    c. acuity increases.
    d. management turnover occurs.

23. A nurse executive wants to decrease the chances of unionization of a non-unionized nursing service department. To accomplish this goal, financial and energy resources would best be directed toward:
    a. increasing nursing salaries and benefits.
    b. improving the overall working conditions for staff, including appointment of highly effective supervisors.
    c. increasing the quality and amount of supplies and equipment.
    d. improving nursing and medical staff relationships.

24. A staff nurse at a unionized agency reports that overtime pay for an after-duty class requiring mandatory attendance was coded as straight pay instead of time and one half as called for in the union contract. Unit managers certify the type and amount of overtime pay. Appropriate action by the nurse executive would be to:
    a. follow up with the nurse's manager to make certain s/he is familiar with the contractual overtime requirements.
    b. accompany the nurse to the payroll office and tell them to make the adjustment.
    c. request that the nurse file a grievance so that payroll adjustment can occur.
    d. turn the matter over to the personnel department for corrective action.

25. Competence of an employee is best determined by:
    a. documentation that the employee meets the requirement of the role.
    b. examination of patient records by a review team.
    c. documentation through a self-administered skills checklist.
    d. evidence of attendance at continuing education courses.

26. The union contract in the facility where you are a manager requires that discipline be progressive in all areas except for substance abuse and theft. Therefore, when an employee commits a first offense of not coming to work as scheduled and neglecting to notify anyone regarding the absence, you would:
    a. give the employee a written reprimand.
    b. counsel the employee verbally (verbal warning).
    c. suspend the employee with pay.
    d. suspend the employee without pay.

27. The planned staffing for 3 South, a 24-bed med-surg unit, calls for a 1:6 staffing ratio (one staff member for each six patients). RNs must comprise 75% of the staff. The unit runs three 8-hour shifts per day, seven days a week, and is generally full to capacity. What is the total number of full time equivalents (FTEs) needed to staff the unit?
    a. 12
    b. 14.4
    c. 16.8
    d. 18.2

28. A labor union is attempting to organize the employees of an institution. It would be considered an unfair labor practice if management:
    a. removed outside organizers from the institution's premises.
    b. refused to allow employees to attend a meeting held by labor organizers during work hours.
    c. supplied the union with information requested about specific employees of the institution.
    d. told employees that the nurse executive would rather deal directly with them than with the union when differences arise.

C

29. The health maintenance organization (HMO) responsible for covering 250,000 lives in a given geographical location does not cover the cost of non-autologous bone marrow transplantation. This therapy is still considered experimental, is rarely successful, and is extremely costly. The ethical principle underlying the HMO's decision is:
    a. beneficence.
    b. autonomy.
    c. justice.
    d. veracity.

30. Despite her family's requests to the contrary, Dr. Huang writes a "Do not resuscitate" order on Mrs. Bosko's chart following a conversation with the patient in which Dr. Huang affirmed the patient's wishes to forgo life-prolonging intervention in the presence of end-stage renal disease. The predominant ethical principle evident in this case is:
    beneficence.
    autonomy.
    justice.
    veracity.

31. Under Title VII of the Civil Rights Act, the employer:
    a. Is not responsible for discrimination on the part of individual supervisors.
    b. Is responsible for discrimination on the part of individual supervisors.
    c. Can terminate a supervisor for practices determined to be discriminatory.
    d. Can sue the individual supervisor to recover monetary loss suffered because of discrimination settlements against the organization because of a supervisor's behavior.

32. A physician who performs a procedure upon a patient without proper consent has committed:
    a. assault.
    b. invasion of privacy.
    c. battery.
    d. false imprisonment.

33. Under Good Samaritan statutes, whoever volunteers to aid another person in distress when the person rendering assistance did not cause the distress assumes:
    a. a legal responsibility to exercise reasonable or ordinary care and skill.
    b. only a moral responsibility to exercise reasonable or ordinary care and skill.
    c. no liability because the person assisting offered that assistance voluntarily.
    d. no legal responsibility to exercise extraordinary care and skill.

34. When an injured person collapses on a jogging path and is discovered by a doctor who is also out jogging, the doctor :
    a. must render necessary emergency treatment on the scene.
    b. must immediately contact emergency services.
    c. has no legal duty to render aid to the injured person.
    d. must provide care under Good Samaritan statutes.

C

35. The physician-patient relationship may be established by:
    a.   an expressed or implied contract.
    b.   a written contract, witnessed and notarized.
    c.   consultation or abandonment.
    d.   punitive damages.

36. When the burden of proof is upon the plaintiff's attorney to show that the plaintiff suffered injury because the defendant violated a legal duty by not following the acceptable standard of care, the case is a:
    a.   malpractice case.
    b.   battery case.
    c.   negligence case.
    d.   defamation case.

37. The individual making a change in a medical record:
    a.   completely erases or otherwise obliterates the original entry.
    b.   destroys the page with the item needing correction and has it redone with the correction completed.
    c.   draws a line through the original entry, leaving it legible, and signs the corrected entry.
    d.   attaches a corrected entry to the record by means of a staple.

38. A physician who specializes in internal medicine, treats a patient for a broken arm. If that patient later brings a suit for malpractice, the physician will be held liable to the standard of care required for:
    a.   his specialty.
    b.   the specialty in which he was treating the patient.
    c.   a general practitioner.
    d.   ordinary medical care.

39. The legal principle that holds the physician liable for the negligence of individuals assisting with a medical procedure is known as:
    a.   res judicata.
    b.   respondeat superior.
    c.   res ipsa loquitor.
    d.   the Captain of the Ship Doctrine.

40. The authority to license health care practitioners is found in the regulating power of:
    a.   the individual hospital.
    b.   the appropriate training program.
    c.   the state.
    d.   the licensing board.

C

41. A nurse executive has staff authority rather than line authority if the nurse executive:
    a. has direct responsibility for accomplishing organizational objectives.
    b. has subordinates over whom authority is exercised.
    c. serves in an advisory capacity.
    d. does not appear on an organizational chart.

42. When developing a mobile health care program for inner-city homeless, the nurse executive considers:
    a. service, cost, and location.
    b. service, cost, and staff mix.
    c. timeframe, cost, and staff mix.
    d. timeframe, location, and service.

43. The nurse has reason to believe that the physician's order is unsafe and refuses to carry it out. Her refusal is made with the knowledge that she:
    a. can be held liable for insubordination.
    b. may be found to be negligent by the state nursing licensing board.
    c. can be held legally accountable for practicing medicine without a license.
    d. can be held liable for any harm that occurs if the order is unsafe but is still carried out by the nurse.

44. With regard to nonprofit institutions, labor-management relations laws, such as the Federal Labor Relations Act:
    a. have no bearing on the relationship between labor and management in non-profit settings.
    b. apply in the nonprofit sector in the same way they apply in the for-profit sector.
    c. are modified for nonprofits as compared with their application in for-profit organizations.
    d. are irrelevant in a unionized organization.

45. The predominant ethical principle underlying the requirements of the Health Insurance Portability and Accountability Act (HIPAA) is that of:
    a. truth-telling (veracity).
    b. confidentiality.
    c. utility.
    d. autonomy.

46. From the perspective of patient rights, the patient whose care is paid for entirely by a third-party entity:
    a. has no right to request an itemized statement of his/her hospital bill.
    b. has the right to request an itemized statement of his/her hospital bill.
    c. may be provided with an itemized statement of his/her hospital bill for a fee.
    d. can obtain the hospital bill only from the third-party payer.

47. In terms of professional ethics, the nurse executive is responsible for ensuring that:
    a. ethics education programs are provided for the nursing staff on an ongoing basis.
    b. a nursing ethics committee is convened and meets regularly.
    c. each nurse in provided with a copy of the Code for Nurses with Interpretive Statements published by the American Nurses Association.
    d. nursing's perspective is represented in the organization's formal mechanisms for addressing ethical dilemmas.

48. The nurse executive's best course of action to stimulate the staff nurses' involvement in research within the organization is to:
    a. hire a well-qualified researcher to conduct research studies.
    b. provide staff nurses with needed time for research activities.
    c. create a joint medical/nursing staff research committee.
    d. ensure that research designs are well grounded and scientific.

49. Which activity is the most important for the nurse executive to personally carry out?
    a. Serve on the policy and procedure committee.
    b. Interpret the job description for a newly hired registered nurse.
    c. Facilitate the dissemination of research in nursing and management systems.
    d. Review the orientation schedule for newly graduated registered nurses.

50. When nurse executives examine job classifications as they plan salary adjustments, they must examine the jobs for equal:
    a. danger on the job, intelligence for hire, and responsibility as well as identical working conditions.
    b. skill, effort, and responsibility as well as similar working conditions.
    c. job requirements, job duties, and equal responsibilities as well as the same working conditions.
    d. effort, working conditions, and equal job requirements as well as identical job duties.

C

Answers to Practice Test

1. a. Incorrect. Rationale: MBO is a collaborative process in which employees establish their own goals rather than relying on managers to set the goals.

   b. Incorrect. Rationale: The collaborative aspect of MBO is not addressed in this response.

   c. Correct. Rationale: Once goals are mutually established, the manager takes on the role of coach as a way of helping the employee meet her goals.

   d. Incorrect. Rationale: The collaborative goals-setting approach is not addressed in this response.

2. a. Correct. Rationale: The organization's philosophy must always be consistent with the mission of the enterprise. In this way there is clarity of intent about what the organization stands for and what it intends to accomplish.

   b. Incorrect. Rationale: Consumer surveys provide important information with regard to the public's perception of the organization and help define the organization's purpose, but survey results are not the main influence with regard to the philosophy of nursing service.

   c. Incorrect. Rationale: Financial resources are used and adjusted to help the organization meet its goals. Financial management flows from the organization's mission and philosophy.

   d. Incorrect. Rationale: Policy development follows and supports the organization's philosophy.

3. a. Correct.   Rationale: Bringing in new talent helps stimulate creativity within the organization and decreases stagnation.

   b. Incorrect.   Rationale: Internal promotion may sustain the status quo rather than stimulating new ideas.

   c. Incorrect.   Rationale: Financial rewards of themselves will not overcome the status quo. Indeed, if people are automatically rewarded for "maintenance," then growth may actually be stymied.

   d. Incorrect.   Rationale: Again, rewarding longevity rather than creativity will sustain the status quo. Stagnation rather than renewal may result.

4. a. Incorrect.   Rationale: While consensus may be desirable, it is not always possible in the face of major change, nor is the change agent necessarily the one to set the parameters of the decision-making process.

   b. Incorrect.   Rationale: Hearing diverse points of view is important to change but is just one step in the process.

   c. Incorrect.   Rationale: This approach thwarts the change agent's effectiveness. The agent's role is to help the group find ways to decrease resistance.

   d. Correct.   Rationale: Unless there is support until the desired change has replaced the status quo, the likelihood of "backsliding" is high. The successful change agent recognizes the need to help her/his clients remain with the process until the desired change has replaced the prior way of doing things.

5. a. Incorrect.   Rationale: Surveys may be used to determine if patient perception is consistent with the marketing strategies in place and to modify the strategy.

   b. Incorrect.   Rationale: Advertising is a marketing technique but should be used only to support what already takes place from the standpoint of patient care.

   c. Correct.   Rationale: The act speaks for itself. From an ethical standpoint, marketing must link to practice. In order to successfully market a specialized service such as oncology, the nurse executive must be confident that the service is of the highest quality. Such an approach prevents false advertising and loss of faith on the part of the public.

d. Incorrect.   Rationale: Hiring an all-licensed staff may or may not be consistent with the marketing strategy for the oncology service.

6. a. Correct.   Rationale: A SWOT analysis helps the organization identify its market share relative to that of its competitors.

    b. Incorrect. Rationale: The risks of over-marketing are not necessarily identified through the needs assessment.

    c. Incorrect. Rationale: The implementation phase of marketing is several steps removed from needs analysis. Certainly the marketing plan will be developed in part based on the needs assessment, but these are two distinct actions.

    d. Incorrect. Rationale: Identifying client needs is also part of the SWOT analysis but is secondary to identifying market share.

7. a. Correct.   Rationale: The basic intent of the decentralized structure is to "push" decision making down as far as is practical to accomplish the goals of the organization and at the same time increase involvement of mid- and first-line managers and staff.

    b. Incorrect. Rationale: Hierarchical decision making is contrary to the philosophy of decentralization.

    c. Incorrect. Rationale: Decentralization is characterized by wide involvement.

    d. Incorrect. Rationale: Decision making in a decentralized organization takes place at the lowest practical level.

8. a. Correct.   Rationale: Evidence-based care trajectories with defined outcomes should be used to effectively and efficiently manage the care of most patients with a given diagnosis or condition.

    b. Incorrect. Rationale: Case managers may be effectively used to accomplish the goals of managed care.

    c. Incorrect. Rationale: The managed care approach assumes commonalties among groups of patients with known diagnoses regardless of the care setting.

    d. Incorrect. Rationale: While each patient is cared for individually, the care given is consistent with a more universal "population-based" approach that applies the law of averages to the care provided.

D

9. a. Incorrect. Rationale: Allowing the group to become distracted and then allowing the subject of the distraction to supplant the main agenda delays needed strategic planning.

    b. Incorrect. Rationale: Staffing problems do not take precedence over strategic planning, which, if done well, may actually alleviate staffing issues downstream.

    c. Correct. Rationale: The chairperson is responsible for keeping the group focused on its purpose and intent consistent with the agreed upon agenda.

    d. Incorrect. Rationale: Each member of the committee makes an important contribution to the work of the group. The need for the presence and engagement of all committee members guarantees that the committee will achieve its intent.

10. a. Incorrect. Rationale: The functional approach focuses on immediate tasks to be accomplished within a short timeframe and within the boundaries of a particular care setting.

    b. Incorrect. Rationale: Primary care nursing is generally confined to a particular setting in which the nurse assumes responsibility for the outcome of care in that setting. The critical path may guide the nurse in the provision of part of the patient's care.

    c. Correct. Rationale: Critical pathways are inherent in the case management approach to care and guide care across the continuum.

    d. Incorrect. Rationale: As with the functional approach, team nursing is concerned primarily with meeting the patient's immediate needs within a particular care setting.

11. a. Incorrect. Rationale: The elimination of staffing problems may or may not be related to a good patient classification system.

    b. Incorrect. Rationale: A decrease in overtime may or may not be related to a good patient classification system.

    c. Correct. Rationale: The purpose of the patient classification system is to predict the category and number of staff members needed to care for a particular patient population.

D

    d.   Incorrect.   Rationale: Patient classification systems should be reviewed periodically to assure they retain their effectiveness in the face of an ever changing environment.

12. a.   Incorrect.   Rationale: Regardless of how efficient or accurate the staffing system, it does not solve the staffing shortages. It may assure that available staff are used in the most productive manner.

    b.   Incorrect.   Rationale: The staffing system may use variable hours depending on its design, the philosophy of the department, and the availability of staff.

    c.   Incorrect.   Rationale: Human error may be reduced or mitigated, but not eliminated, by the use of a good classification system.

    d.   Correct.   Rationale: The dynamic nature of health care, changing patient characteristics, the introduction of new technology, and so forth requires that nursing departments episodically review the current patient classification process.

13. a.   Correct.   Rationale: The underlying philosophy of TQM is a focus on the customer/client as the reason for taking action to improve quality.

    b.   Incorrect.   Rationale: Analysis of processes and systems and making process changes is key to the success of TQM.

    c.   Incorrect.   Rationale: TQM puts the client at the center of the process. The organization exists to serve its customers.

    d.   Incorrect.   Rationale: Efficiency and cost containment may result from application of the TQM process, but this concept is not the predominant principle.

14. a.   Correct.   Rationale: Congruency between the organization's mission, vision, philosophy, goals, and objectives is essential to the success of the entity.

    b.   Incorrect.   Rationale: Philosophy is an intangible guide. In the strict sense of the word, it is not quantifiable.

    c.   Incorrect.   Rationale: Goals flow from mission and philosophy.

    d.   Incorrect.   Rationale: While it is desirable for the philosophy to be well understood, brevity is less important than meaning or congruency with the organization's mission and vision.

D

15. a. Correct.   Rationale: Satisfaction survey information is considered qualitative. Satisfaction is based on perception and as such is subjective.

　　b. Incorrect.   Rationale: Quantitative measure.

　　c. Incorrect.   Rationale: Quantitative measure.

　　d. Incorrect.   Rationale: Quantitative measure.

16. a. Correct.   Rationale: This approach demonstrates compliance with basic accounting principles and makes explicit the department's fiduciary accountability.

　　b. Incorrect.   Rationale: Timely submission of budgets is a process expectation.

　　c. Incorrect.   Rationale: This activity may be a process expectation within the organization.

　　d. Incorrect.   Rationale: This is an expectation consistent with principles of business ethics, but of itself is not sufficient to demonstrate full accountability.

17. a. Incorrect.   Rationale: Incorrect calculation.

　　b. Correct.   Rationale: Correct calculation: $1.4 million x .80 = $1.12 million.

　　c. Incorrect.   Rationale: Incorrect calculation.

　　d. Incorrect.   Rationale: Incorrect calculation.

18. a. Incorrect.   Rationale: Incorrect calculation.

　　b. Correct.   Rationale: Calculation: $1.6 million x .85 = $1.36 million.

　　c. Incorrect.   Rationale: Incorrect calculation.

　　d. Incorrect.   Rationale: Incorrect calculation.

19. a. Incorrect.   Rationale: Calculation: $1.6 million x .15 = $240,000 x .90 = $216,000.

　　b. Incorrect.   Rationale: Incorrect calculation.

　　c. Incorrect.   Rationale: Incorrect calculation.

　　d. Incorrect.   Rationale: Incorrect calculation.

D

20. a.   Incorrect.   Rationale: While it is important for staff to understand the ramifications of cost containment, education alone will not result in cost reduction.

   b.   Correct.   Rationale: By knowing the specific cost of care of various patient categories, the nurse executive, along with others within the department, has needed knowl edge upon which to base a cost-containment plan.

   c.   Incorrect.   Rationale: Cost shifting will not help the organization reduce its overall costs.

   d.   Incorrect.   Rationale: While increased involvement by nursing in the governance of the organization is a worthy objective, baseline data is still needed in order to measure the effectiveness of any cost-reduction strategies.

21. a.   Correct.   Rationale: Provides needed data for accurate financial reporting and comparison.

   b.   Incorrect.   Rationale: Patient care requirements are included as part of creating the nursing workload system. Physician recommendations may be taken into consideration, but this step is not essential in fiscal oversight for the nursing department budget.

   c.   Incorrect.   Rationale: Provides needed but insufficient data.

   d.   Incorrect.   Rationale: May indirectly contribute to fiscal stability.

22. a.   Correct.   Rationale: This model is based on the premise that a certain volume is needed to maintain cost balance. When the volume decreases below the break-even point, costs go up. For example, staffing for a 50-bed unit is calculated for an occupancy rate of 85% with a break-even point of 80%. Downward adjustments in staff numbers occur only when the occupancy rate dips to 75%. Any occupancy rate between 76 and 79% results in a "loss" based on the cost model.

   b.   Incorrect.   Rationale: An increase in volume does not necessarily translate to an increase in cost per unit of service.

   c.   Incorrect.   Rationale: This may or may not be an accurate statement. Increased acuity does not necessarily equate to an increase in cost per unit of service.

   d.   Incorrect.   Rationale: Management turnover should not impact cost per unit of service.

D

23. a.   Incorrect.   Rationale: Assuring that salaries and benefits are comparable to those in unionized facilities is an important step, but, of itself, is not sufficient to forestall unionization activities.

   b.   Correct.   Rationale: Discontent with working conditions and management conflict are among the greatest dissatisfiers for staff. Improving overall working conditions and assuring the presence of a highly skilled, sensitive managerial staff may lessen the possibility of unionization.

   c.   Incorrect.   Rationale: Such an intervention may be of help, but, of itself, it is not sufficient to forestall union organizing activities.

   d.   Incorrect.   Rationale: While important of itself, this is an insufficient intervention to lessen the possibility of unionization.

24. a.   Correct.   Rationale: Managers are responsible for knowing the legalities and contract requirements regarding overtime. By encouraging the manager to become more familiar with the contract, the nurse executive helps the manager fulfill her/his responsibilities and adds to the manager's competency.

   b.   Incorrect.   Rationale: This is not an executive-level function.

   c.   Incorrect.   Rationale: The issue can be successfully resolved without resorting to the grievance procedure. In addition, management cannot place itself in the position of encouraging anyone to file a grievance.

   d.   Incorrect.   Rationale: Resolution of the issue should be handled at the appropriate level by the employee's manager. There is no reason to involve the personnel department in this case.

25. a.   Correct.   Rationale: The employee's competence is verified through observation and review of objective data and then documented. Documentation of competence to per form a particular job is an external regulatory and internal policy requirement.

   b.   Incorrect.   Rationale: Review of records is may be part of competency verification, but, of itself, is insufficient to determine competence.

c. Incorrect. Rationale: Self assessment is also an aid in determining competence but cannot stand alone as the sole mechanism for verifying competence.

d. Incorrect. Rationale: Continuing education may contribute to enhancement of employee competence but cannot be directly correlated with the employee's level of competence.

26. a. Incorrect. Rationale: A written warning is generally the second step in the progressive discipline process.

b. Correct. Rationale: The first action by the manager in the progressive discipline process is a verbal warning.

c. Incorrect. Rationale: Suspension with or without pay are subsequent steps in the progressive discipline process.

d. Incorrect. Rationale: In some union environments, suspension without pay is prohibited by contract.

27. a. Incorrect. Rationale: Incorrect/incomplete calculation.

b. Incorrect. Rationale: Incorrect calculation.

c. Correct. Rationale: Four staff members per 8-hour shift are required to care for 24 patients around the clock. Four staff members x 3 shifts = 12 employees. The unit operates seven days a week, thus 1.4 FTEs per position are needed to meet the needs of the unit. 12 x 1.4 = 16.8.

d. Incorrect. Rationale: Incorrect calculation.

28. a. Incorrect. Rationale: This action is within the rights of management.

b. Incorrect. Rationale: This action is within the rights of management.

c. Correct. Rationale: This action is contrary to regulations governing collective bargaining activities.

d. Incorrect. Rationale: This action is within the rights of management. It is generally considered a political move on the part of management.

D

29. a. Incorrect. Rationale: Beneficence suggests that the treatment, regardless of its efficacy, should be offered (or withheld) for the good of the patient as determined by her/his agent (usually the physician). The decision is made without regard to the impact it may have on others.

  b. Incorrect. Rationale: Autonomy implies that the patient has a "right" to self-determination and, as such, has a right to experimental treatment.

  c. Correct. Rationale: The principle of distributive justice, as applied in the HMO setting, holds that those interventions that can do the most good for the greatest number are the interventions that should be offered, particularly because there is no way for the organization to recover "extraordinary" costs given its funding constraints. To offer a costly, unproven therapy to one member of the HMO plan exposes the organization to jeopardy in that it may then be impelled to offer the same intervention to all.

  d. Incorrect. Rationale: Assuring that the patient has a truthful explanation of the benefits and burdens of any treatment honors the principle of truth-telling. However, veracity is not the pivotal principle in this case.

30. a. Incorrect. Rationale: Beneficence holds that others, primarily the physician, are responsible for making decisions on the patient's behalf. In this case, beneficence and autonomy may be seen as complementary to one another, assuming that the decision the patient has made on her own behalf is consistent with the decision the physician would have made about her care in any case.

  b. Correct. Rationale: Autonomy holds that the patient's wishes are to be respected even of her wishes are contrary to those of her family. The covenant is between patient and physician. In this case, the physician honors the patient's decision. The patient's competence to make decisions about the extent of her care is not in question.

  c. Incorrect. Rationale: Not the predominant principle in this case.

  d. Incorrect. Rationale: Not the predominant principle in this case.

31. a. Incorrect. Rationale: Not true. The act holds the employer responsible for the acts of its employees.

D

b. Correct.   Rationale: This statement is true. The act stipulates that the employer remains responsible for the acts of its employees.

c. Incorrect. Rationale: Though a supervisor may be terminated because of discriminatory acts, such action is not a requirement of Title VII.

d. Incorrect. Rationale: Though an employer can attempt to recover loss in this way, Title VII includes no stipulation with regard to such recovery.

32. a. Incorrect. Rationale: Assault is defined as "knowingly threatening another."

b. Incorrect. Rationale: Invasion of privacy means the "disclosure of personal information considered to be confidential or intrusion in a situation where there is a reasonable expectation of privacy."

c. Correct.   Rationale: Except in an emergency situation, where consent is implied, the performance of a procedure upon a patient without his/her explicit consent, or the explicit consent of his/her agent where indicated, constitutes battery on the part of the practitioner. Battery is defined as "the deliberate touching of another without authorization."

d. Incorrect. Rationale: False imprisonment means the unlawful restraint of an individual's personal liberty.

33. a. Correct.   Rationale: Those who elect to provide assistance in the presence of an unforeseen emergency are held to the ordinary standard of skill, competence, and judgment expected of a reasonably prudent person with the same preparation.

b. Incorrect. Rationale: Legal responsibility, as well as moral responsibility, is assumed under Good Samaritan statutes.

c. Incorrect. Rationale: There is an exemption from liability because of the emergency nature of the situation, not because of the voluntary nature of the situation.

d. Incorrect. Rationale: The legal responsibility under the Good Samaritan statute is to exercise ordinary care and skill.

34. a. Incorrect. Rationale: The physician is under no obligation to render treatment.

D

b. Incorrect. Rationale: One assumes a reasonable person coming upon an emergency situation will contact emergency services (911), though there is no absolute obligation to do so.

c. Correct. Rationale: The physician is not impelled by law to render aid to the person who has collapsed.

d. Incorrect. Rationale: Good Samaritan legislation offers protection to those who voluntarily assist in an emergency situation. It does not compel anyone to offer such care.

35. a. Correct. Rationale: The fact that the patient seeks care, or, in the case of an emergency, needs care, can be interpreted as an implied contract.

b. Incorrect. Rationale: Such an approach is not considered standard or common practice.

c. Incorrect. Rationale: The physician may enter into the patient's care through consultation or because another physician has inappropriately abandoned the case, but this is not the usual mechanism through which the physician-patient relationship is established.

d. Incorrect. Rationale: Not the basis for a physician-patient relationship.

36. a. Correct. Rationale: The case as presented suggests that the elements needed to satisfy a charge of malpractice may well exist. These elements are duty (to practice to a known and accepted standard), breach of duty, causation, and injury.

b. Incorrect. Rationale: Whether or not battery occurred cannot be determined from the situation as presented.

c. Incorrect. Rationale: Negligence implies that the failure to perform in accordance with what a reasonable person would do was unintentional. In this case, the plaintiff's attorney will attempt to show that harm was intentional.

d. Incorrect. Rationale: Whether or not defamation is involved in this case cannot be determined from the situation as presented. Defamation does not appear to be a factor in the case.

D

37. a. Incorrect. Rationale: Original chart entries are never to be obliterated.

   b. Incorrect. Rationale: Original chart pages are never to be destroyed.

   c. Correct. Rationale: This is the long-accepted procedure for correcting documentation errors in the medical record.

   d. Incorrect. Rationale: There must be an indication that the original entry was incorrect. Stapling the corrected entry to the original entry is not advised.

38. a. Incorrect. Rationale: If the physician presumes to treat, then s/he must treat according to the needs of the patient as established by standards within a specialty.

   b. Correct. Rationale: The patient can reasonably expect that his broken bone will be set according to the standards of orthopedic practice. If the internal medicine physician cannot perform to this standard, then s/he should assure that the care of the patient is transferred to someone who can practice accordingly.

   c. Incorrect. Rationale: See above.

   d. Incorrect. Rationale: An essentually meaningless term.

39. a. Incorrect. Rationale: Res judica applies to the final judgment in a case.

   b. Incorrect. Rationale: Respondeat superior applies to the responsibility an organization has for the actions of its employees or staff.

   c. Incorrect. Rationale: Res ipsa loquitor means "the thing speaks for itself" and also may apply in this case, but not as specifically as the Captain of the Ship Doctrine.

   d. Correct. Rationale: Because of the physician's unique status and expertise, s/he may be held liable for the actions of those who assist with a medical (usually a surgical) procedure.

40. a. Incorrect. Rationale: There is no such thing as institutional licensure.

   b. Incorrect. Rationale: Training programs prepare personnel for licensure, they do not issue licenses.

   c. Correct. Rationale: The state issues regulations pertaining to licensure of various professions.

   d. Incorrect. Rationale: The licensing board is charged by the state to issue the license. However, it is the state, not the licensing board, that regulates licensure.

D

41. a. Incorrect. Rationale: Implies line authority.

    b. Incorrect. Rationale: Implies line authority.

    c. Correct. Rationale: With no direct reports and no absolute account-ability for achieving organizational goals, the executive in this case has staff authority. Even so, s/he may hold influential or expert power and be able to effect significant organizational change even without line authority.

    d. Incorrect. Rationale: It is appropriate for such a person to appear on the organizational chart and organizational chart protocol assures a method for doing so.

42. a. Correct. Rationale: Service, cost, and location are first-order priorities. Other elements flow from them. For example, staff mix can be established once services and cost (or investment) are known.

    b. Incorrect. Rationale: All elements are important. As noted above, staff mix in this case is not considered a first-level priority.

    c. Incorrect. Rationale: The timeframe can be established only after the location, cost, and service are known.

    d. Incorrect. Rationale: The critical element of cost is missing in this list.

43. a. Incorrect. Rationale: The nurse is not liable for insubordination in that s/he took action in the best interest of the patient based on her/his professional knowledge and judgment.

    b. Incorrect. Rationale: The nurse may be found liable if s/he carries out the order and such action results in harm to the patient.

    c. Incorrect. Rationale: In the scenario presented, the nurse is acting consistent with the requirements of her/his profession. Nothing in the statement suggests that the nurse is "practicing medicine."

D

d.   Correct.   Rationale: The nurse has a obligation to know and understand the risks, benefits, and boundaries of interventions ordered by the physician. Should the order be deemed inaccurate or incorrect, the nurse can be held liable if s/he carries out the order. The expectation on the part of the nurse is that s/he will question, clarify, and, when necessary, refuse to carry out an order that may cause harm to the patient.

44. a.   Incorrect.   Rationale: Labor-management relations laws apply equally in for-profit and not-for-profit settings.

b.   Correct.   Rationale: This is an accurate statement.

c.   Incorrect.   Rationale: The laws are not modified according to the organization's profit status.

d.   Incorrect.   Rationale: The laws apply in a union enviroment as well as in a non-union environment.

45. a.   Incorrect.   Rationale: HIPAA promises full and accurate disclosure about the manner in which personal health information is used and shared. Thus, veracity can be seen as applicable to HIPAA. However, confidentiality is the predominant principle underlying the intent of HIPAA.

b.   Correct.   Rationale: HIPAA promises stringent adherence to the principles of confidentiality and includes stiff penalties in the face of violation of its tenets.

c.   Incorrect.   Rationale: Not the predominant principle underlying HIPAA.

d.   Incorrect.   Rationale: Not the predominant principle underlying HIPAA.

46. a.   Incorrect.   Rationale: The method of payment has no bearing on the patient's right to request an itemized bill from the hospital.

b.   Correct.   Rationale: The patient has a right to obtain a statement of his/her hospital bill regardless of how the hospital bill is paid.

c.   Incorrect.   Rationale: There is no fee attached to obtaining an itemized bill of the patient's hospital stay.

d.   Incorrect.   Rationale: There is no such restriction.

D

47. a. Incorrect. Rationale: While ethics education is certainly of benefit to nurses, the nurse executive is under no obligation to guarantee that such education is offered by the institution.

    b. Incorrect. Rationale: Whether or not an organization convenes a nursing ethics committee in addition to the multidisciplinary ethics committee in place in acute care facilities is a decision driven by organizational intent. It is not a requirement.

    c. Incorrect. Rationale: While providing nurses with a copy of the Code for Nurses speaks to the professionalism of the executive team, assuring that each nurse has a copy of the code is not a mandate.

    d. Correct. Rationale: The nurse executive assures that nursing is well represented within whatever formal framework the organization has in place to deal with ethical issues. Nursing is generally represented on the organization's multidisciplinary ethics committee. Policies and procedures are in place to guide nurses faced with ethical dilemmas in the course of their practice.

48. a. Incorrect. Rationale: A highly qualified researcher may be of great value to the organization's intent to involve staff nurses in research activities if her/his skills are directed toward helping staff nurses design their own research projects.

    b. Correct. Rationale: If research at the staff nurse level is a value of the organization, the organization will find a way to provide the staff with time to engage in research activities.

    c. Incorrect. Rationale: Such a committee may support the research efforts but, of itself, will not achieve the goal of involvement of staff in actual research.

    d. Incorrect. Rationale: This is an important part of the learning process as staff nurses take on the role of researchers. By itself, knowledge of proper research design does not translate to increased involvement by staff nurses in the research process.

49. a. Incorrect. Rationale: The nurse executive should assure adequate representation on the policy and procedure committee and delegate responsibility for management of the committee to a subordinate.

    b. Incorrect. Rationale: This is a managerial and human resources function. It is not an executive-level function.

    c. Correct. Rationale: Such an activity is within the purview of the executive. By assuring systems are in place to disseminate research in both nursing and management, the nurse executive helps set expectations for the organization's leadership group.

    d. Incorrect. Rationale: This is a managerial function, not an executive-level function.

50. a. Incorrect. Rationale: Inaccurate requirements under the equal-pay test. In particular, intelligence testing is implied, but is not required. The intent of the equal-pay test is to check for comparable, not identical, conditions.

    b. Correct. Rationale: This statement accurately reflects the equal-pay test requirements.

    c. Incorrect. Rationale: Partially correct only.

    d. Incorrect. Rationale: Partially correct only.

D

Index

3